D0975751

NO LONGER PROPERTY
OF ANYTHINK
RANGEVIEW LIBRARY
DISTRICT

# THE
# ALL-DAY
# FAT-BURNING
# DIET

# THE
# ALL-DAY
# FAT-BURNING
# DIET

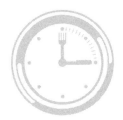

### The 5-Day Food-Cycling Formula
### That Resets Your Metabolism to
### LOSE UP TO 5 POUNDS A WEEK

# YURI ELKAIM

### *New York Times* bestselling author of
### *The All-Day Energy Diet*

RODALE.

# RODALE *wellness*

*Live happy. Be healthy. Get inspired.*

Sign up today to get exclusive access to our authors, exclusive bonuses, and the most authoritative, useful, and cutting-edge information on health, wellness, fitness, and living your life to the fullest.
**Visit us online at RodaleWellness.com**
**Join us at RodaleWellness.com/Join**

---

This book is intended as a reference volume only, not as a medical manual. The information given here is designed to help you make informed decisions about your health. It is not intended as a substitute for any treatment that may have been prescribed by your doctor. If you suspect that you have a medical problem, we urge you to seek competent medical help.

The information in this book is meant to supplement, not replace, proper exercise training. All forms of exercise pose some inherent risks. The editors and publisher advise readers to take full responsibility for their safety and know their limits. Before practicing the exercises in this book, be sure that your equipment is well-maintained, and do not take risks beyond your level of experience, aptitude, training, and fitness. The exercise and dietary programs in this book are not intended as a substitute for any exercise routine or dietary regimen that may have been prescribed by your doctor. As with all exercise and dietary programs, you should get your doctor's approval before beginning.

Mention of specific companies, organizations, or authorities in this book does not imply endorsement by the author or publisher, nor does mention of specific companies, organizations, or authorities imply that they endorse this book, its author, or the publisher.

Internet addresses and telephone numbers given in this book were accurate at the time it went to press.

© 2015 by Yuri Elkaim and Elkaim Group International, Inc.

All rights reserved. No part of this publication may be reproduced or transmitted in any form or by any means, electronic or mechanical, including photocopying, recording, or any other information storage and retrieval system, without the written permission of the publisher.

Rodale books may be purchased for business or promotional use or for special sales. For information, please write to:
Special Markets Department, Rodale Inc., 733 Third Avenue, New York, NY 10017

Printed in the United States of America
Rodale Inc. makes every effort to use acid-free ♾, recycled paper ♻.

Illustrations by Jason Lee
Book design by Amy C. King

Library of Congress Cataloging-in-Publication Data is on file with the publisher.

ISBN 978–1–62336–605–6

Distributed to the trade by Macmillan

2  4  6  8  10  9  7  5  3     hardcover

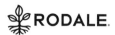

---

We inspire and enable people to improve their lives and the world around them.
rodalebooks.com

*Dedicated to my wife, Amy, for giving me the extra nudge
at 5 a.m. each day to write this book . . .
and to Oscar, Luca, and Arlo for making it necessary
to get up that early. I love you guys.*

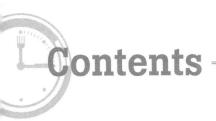

# Contents

# Mission Statement

The reason I wrote this book is simple: Despite all the attempts we've made as a society over the past 50 years to get slimmer and improve our health, we've accomplished almost the complete opposite. Today, many people are frustrated with repeated weight loss (and weight regain), diet failures, and a chronic inability to look and feel the way they want. You might be one of them.

I want you to know that it's not your fault. You've been raised in a world characterized by confusing information, conflicting advice, and man-made foods that wreak havoc on your body. So much of this is out of your hands, so please don't beat yourself up over it. With the sound information and the proven plan you now have in your hands, you can make a change. The ball is in your court.

I can show the way to the promised land, but you have to do the walking. You have to put in the work. I'll be with you each step of the way, but I need you to make a decision that you're in. All change happens in a split second. And it happens when you make a decision. If you're sick and tired of struggling with your weight and feel you deserve better (because you do), then make a decision right now to commit to following my lead.

All I'm asking is that you follow my plan for the next 21 days. Can you do that with me?

Believe me, I understand that change is uncomfortable. It's the last thing we humans want to do. But to get the body you want, you can't just dabble. You have to commit. You need to master yourself, your diet, and your habits. That's what I'm here to help you accomplish with this book.

For the past 15 years, I've helped more than 500,000 people achieve their health and fitness goals. My mission is to help 10 million people by 2018 and 100 million by 2024. Yes, I'm on a pretty ambitious mission, but I have no doubt that I'll accomplish these goals.

My unique ability lies in how I simplify people's lives by erasing the complexity from diet and fitness, boiling them down to simple, tangible action steps that give people a principle-based understanding of their health. In this book, you'll have many aha moments as I dispel a number of health myths—especially diet and exercise myths—and give you easy-to-follow advice and a 21-day plan that doesn't require counting calories, depriving yourself, or killing yourself in the gym.

If you've been told that eating less and exercising more are the keys to losing weight and you've tried multiple diets with temporary success and ultimate failure, then this book is the solution you've been looking for. Why? Because my plan eliminates the causes of weight gain and pushes the reset button on your fat-burning capacity. And it does so in a way that also improves your health.

Yes, you'll experience quick weight loss. And yes, this weight loss will likely last longer than ever before. The reason is that we're going to provide your body with a plan that will help restore it to its "factory setting"—one where it's primed to burn fat, not store it. Very few people understand the real causes of stubborn weight gain. Here's the secret: Your body is set to either gain, maintain, or lose weight all day, and no combination of calorie cutting, exercising, or restrictive dieting will help you look and feel great unless you reset your body to burn fat and lose weight on autopilot.

Let me show you how.

# Introduction

## *I Feel Your Pain*

As a child and young man, Adam never really knew what it meant to be slim, fit, or even reasonably happy. For nearly 20 years of his life, he struggled with his weight and was mercilessly teased by his friends and even his older brother for being so chubby. There was no limit to the names they called him, and he was often the last kid picked in gym class to join a team. He thought this misery was normal.

What's strange was that Adam didn't eat much differently than his skinny brother, nor did he eat a great deal more. They both feasted regularly on the same amount of junk food—hot dogs, microwave dinners, grilled cheese sandwiches, chocolate bars, and plenty of upsized, cholesterol-laden specials from far too many drive-thru windows. Neither of his parents was overweight, nor were his grandparents.

What could account for Adam's girth? Was he just born that way and destined to remain hefty as long as he lived? Why was it such a struggle for him to lose even a pound while his brother seemed genetically programmed to be skinny no matter how much crap he ate? Before I answer that question, I have a confession: Tubby little Adam was my brother. I was the wicked, skinny brother.

You're certainly familiar with my type; you've seen me in several Disney movies—that mean, slender grouch who is constantly picking on his pudgy, gentle sidekick. That was the two of us, and I was unrelenting. I bossed him around, belittled him whenever I could, and forced him to play soccer and road hockey with me even when he didn't want to. I was awful.

As much as it hurts to say this, and even though I've changed, I was a bully—at least to him. Mocking him and making him do my bidding was a sport to me, and I didn't fully understand just how much my taunting and teasing hurt him on the inside. I'd like to believe that if I'd known, I would've stopped, but that's hard to say. Thankfully, the universe has a funny way of evening the score, as you've no doubt seen in those same Disney movies I mentioned. Eventually, our terrible diet caught up with me as well, and though I didn't put on an inch of fat, I'd end up suffering just as much as Adam did.

One evening, just a few days before my 17th birthday, I hopped into the shower after a particularly draining soccer practice. As I ran my fingers through my flowing brown hair, a sense of calm washed over me. Then, I looked at my hands. Both of my palms were streaked with thick clumps of my hair. Panicked, I touched my head, only for more to come off in my hands. What was happening to me? I could barely get to sleep that night, but when I finally did, I soon woke up to a real-life nightmare. My pillow was covered in hair. In less than 6 weeks, I would lose all of my hair—even my eyelashes. I was completely bald from head to toe.

I walked through the halls of my high school with all eyes trained on my shiny new head. Without eyelashes or eyebrows, I looked like an alien fit to be dissected in the biology lab. People jeered, stared, and laughed. Many people stayed as far away from me as possible. They wondered if what I had was contagious. This was my senior year of high school, when I was just about to set foot into the world of adulthood. I was crushed, scared, and confused. There was nowhere I could hide.

This was far worse than male-pattern baldness; this was something else. My immunologist told me that I had an autoimmune condition called alopecia. However, he had no answers beyond that diagnosis: Why did it happen? He didn't know. What could I do? He didn't know. And after 7 painstaking years of dealing with the medical community, I came to realize that most doctors didn't know either. No matter what type of specialist I consulted, not a single doctor had any idea what to do other than to inject cortisone directly into my scalp. Not once did any of these general practitioners or specialists ever speculate what may have caused my health problems or what could be done to permanently solve them. They were more interested in getting me on experimental pills or steroid creams or injecting my scalp with who knows what. By the time I was 24 years old, I was fed up. My frustration led to a life-changing decision.

Realizing that our "health care" system was not going to help me get back to better health, I vowed to crawl under every rock and read every book I could, if necessary, to figure out what was wrong with me. If no one could give me any answers, I was going to find them myself. I would be the source of my own healing.

First came 4 years of study at the University of Toronto, from which I graduated with a degree in physical education and health/kinesiology. I didn't view this as a great accomplishment, though, as I still hadn't grasped how to truly be healthy. My next step was to enroll at a natural nutrition school. It was there that I learned that my autoimmune disorder and other health issues were greatly related to years of dietary abuse. My athleticism was of little consequence; I was rotting from the inside out.

I made a decision to set my body on a healthier course, and with that, I ditched several foods from my diet. Within a few short months, I was feeling my old energy return; moreover, most of my hair had grown back. My digestive problems, eczema, and breathing problems vanished as well.

You might be wondering what, if anything, this has to do with weight loss. What I came to learn during this harrowing period is that our health is far more dependent on our diet than we've been led to believe. An unhealthy diet can manifest itself in all kinds of ways. I believe it caused me to lose my hair and, more insidiously, led to my suffering from chronically low energy, a condition that I addressed in my first book, *The All-Day Energy Diet*. In this book, I'll take a look at how our awful eating habits and other lifestyle decisions flip on the fat-gain switch in our bodies. This is a trend I've personally witnessed in my work helping thousands of personal clients and more than half a million online clients and viewers develop lean, fit, and healthy bodies over the past 2 decades. Although low energy levels and fat gain arise from the same origin, they require different fixes.

In the chapters to come, I'll share the strategy I developed from my personal experience and investigations into health to help thousands of people around the world shut off that fat-gaining switch for good and reset their metabolism to burn fat 24/7. In case you're wondering, my brother Adam is one of them. I had to atone for my sins, and it really was a joy to share all that I learned with him so he could overhaul his life. Today, he's slimmer and taller than I am. We've worked together for years to help him attain the body he's always wanted, and his becoming a part of my health business has been a major catalyst toward this goal.

Adam's success has been rewarding for us both, but unfortunately my journey to good health had yet another chapter that is relevant to your weight-loss mission.

My recovery and new education gave me the basis for a successful Internet business through which I've helped people all over the world. My videos have earned more than 15 million views on YouTube, and I've published a *New York Times* bestselling book. I was living the dream, but it meant nothing to me when I lost my eyebrows . . . again.

You can't imagine the fear I felt. What was happening to me? Did this mean there was no truth to what I was teaching? Flooded with fears of my alopecia returning and my business falling apart, I did what any grown man would do: I started secretly using my wife's makeup to fill in my thinning eyebrows.

The shedding increased and I developed a makeup routine, applying my fake eyebrows every morning after I brushed my teeth. I eventually started toning down my workouts out of fear that my sweat would make my "eyebrows" run. I refused to go swimming with my kids because the water might ruin my makeup. I continued shooting and posting YouTube videos but was in constant fear of being outed as a fraud. It was exhausting.

In late 2013, I went to a 4-day personal and business development event in the Dominican Republic. I had no idea what to expect, but I was certainly meant to be there because it profoundly affected my life—for the better. After the first 2 days, I sat down one evening to catch up with my friend Dane. As we so often do, we had a long conversation about what was happening in our lives. That's when everything came spilling out. I opened up about everything I was dealing with: my eyebrows, the makeup, and why I was afraid. I don't think I had ever been this vulnerable or open about my feelings. Being the amazing person that he is, Dane peered into my soul and worked some kind of magic that touched me at a fundamental level. Something shifted inside of me.

Later that evening, I was having another conversation with a good friend, Fabienne, whom I hadn't seen for about a year. We were talking about one of the exercises from the event in which we were asked to give away something of value to us. Most people had brought jewelry and other personal mementos. I couldn't think of anything to bring that was meaningful to me—other than my children. I didn't think it would be wise to give them away! Then, it hit me. There was only one thing I was holding on to like a baby does a blankie. Any ideas? Take a guess. It was that damn eyebrow makeup. Could I really get rid of it? Could I take off the mask and bare my true self? Deep down inside, I knew the answer.

That evening's conversation with Fabienne reaffirmed my belief that this was the right thing to do. She reassured me that I was a beautiful person and gave me the courage I needed to take the leap. I broke down in front of her. I couldn't keep up my disguise any longer. I promised Fabienne that the next morning I would be done with the makeup for good, and because my word means everything to me, that's exactly what happened. The next morning, I walked straight into the bathroom, picked up the makeup, and chucked it into the trash can. I stared in the mirror at the shiny patches of flesh above my eyes. There was no turning back now.

Anxiously, I left my hotel room and made my way to the beach for a morning yoga session. I felt naked and awkward and kept glancing around to see who was looking at me. Oddly enough, no one really noticed. I felt weird, but then, it wasn't like I was wearing a giant scarlet letter *A* on my chest. What happened next was pure magic. As I moved through each position in our yoga session, my body was soothed by the warm morning sun. About halfway through the session, it started raining, even while the sun was shining. I remember lying on my mat with my eyes closed and relishing the feeling of the warm rain splashing my face.

After the yoga session, I ran to the ocean with childlike excitement, crashing through the waves and diving headfirst into the salty water. As I swam underwater, time froze. It was like living in slow motion. When I surfaced, I wiped the water off my face, opened my eyes, and felt more alive than ever before. I was finally free. I felt like I'd just baptized myself in a sense. My true self had finally emerged. I reflected on the fact that all life initially came from the ocean, so it was fitting that, with my first step out of the water, I felt reborn.

For nearly 2 years, I had hidden underneath a mask of shame, worrying about what people would think of me if I shared my struggle. The irony is that I felt more free, more happy, and more alive without the makeup than I ever did when I was wearing it. As painful as it is to relive these memories, I share this story for this reason: If you've ever felt ashamed about your weight or how you look, then believe me, I've been there. I can totally relate, and this is a big part of why I was inspired to write this book. Having gone through intense shame and disgust with myself, I came to understand what Adam must have felt all those years ago when I was unrelenting in my teasing. I can only imagine how you feel, not so happy with how you look in the mirror, always self-conscious about how others see you. I want you to find the relief and self-love that both Adam and I have found.

If you want to lose 20 pounds, that's great. You should. Being a fit and healthy person is important. You'll feel better about yourself for doing what needs to be done to get you there. But start now by showing yourself a little compassion. As you're about to find out in the next chapter, being overweight is largely no fault of your own. That's right—you can stop blaming yourself so much.

By easing up on yourself, you'll likely experience a pleasant surprise: People are far more accepting of you when you're accepting of yourself. Upon my return from the trip, I shot a video for my audience in which, for the first time ever, I was makeup free. This was easily the scariest moment of my life, putting myself out there for potentially millions of people to eventually see, but I wanted to come clean. What happened next continues to touch me deeply: Within minutes of my posting it, tons of comments started pouring in from viewers and clients who thanked me for being real and honest with them and giving them permission to be and love themselves. I felt a new peace, and it's ultimately what I want for you as well. (To this day, that video is still online. It's called "My Coming Out—Part 2," and you can check it out if you like.)

The goal of this book, helping you lose up to 5 pounds per week with my proven 5-Day Food-Cycling Formula, may strike you as superficial. But it's really about allowing you to be your true self, freeing you of the shackles that have held you back for far too long. I want to strip away the complexity and confusion and make your life a whole lot easier by giving you a proven, very intuitive plan. It's something you can practice for the rest of your life if you want to. This plan jibes with the way your body has been hardwired since the beginning of time. It craves for you to give it what it needs. I hope you're ready to do so!

I've worked with enough people in the last 2 decades to know that no one, not a single person, in spite of what he says, feels good when he's overweight. Let's be honest—we are all motivated by vanity. We all want to look better. And we totally should. That's part of striving to be a better version of ourselves. When you look good, you feel good. And when you feel good, you look even better. I know you can do that without plastic surgery or radical quick fixes.

Over the course of this book and the 3 weeks to follow (and hopefully beyond), we'll be deconstructing all of the ways we inadvertently allow our bodies to pack on the pounds—from what we eat for breakfast to what we do before we go to bed every night. We'll pick apart your diet and replace the junk you may have been eating with nourishing and delicious foods that reset your metabolism and allow you to burn fat more easily. We will not only address what meals you should eat, but how and when to eat them, as these meals will be the heart of the 5-Day Food-Cycling Formula.

In Chapter 10, I'll give you the exact meal plan to follow for your first 21 days, along with all the recipes you'll need. This is the same plan that has yielded the amazing transformations you'll read about in this book. I chose 21 days because that's a great starting point for creating lasting habits, but you'll likely find that you can sustain this lifestyle much longer.

Why is food cycling so important for losing weight? Well, up until the last 100 years, humans didn't have the luxury of eating five or six meals per day. Nor were their meals bombarded with the chemicals and toxins that are a mainstay in today's food supply. Our early ancestors thrived on oscillating periods of feasting, fasting, and grazing on fresh foods found in nature. Yet today we mistakenly believe that eating every 2 or 3 hours keeps our metabolism "revved up" and that man-made, synthetic foods are the most convenient way to nourish ourselves. Obviously, our waistlines and health have paid the price—big time. As you'll discover in the next chapter, there are six reasons why the modern world has made us fatter than ever. These six "fat triggers" shift our metabolisms and upset the normal hormone function inside our bodies, causing us to gain and hold on to fat. Everything in this book is built around rectifying those six fat triggers so that you can lose weight for good.

Finally, we'll address your body both at rest and at work—from how to properly recharge your body to how you can develop an efficient and enjoyable workout schedule that powers you up and turns you into a lean, fat-burning machine.

The goal is simple: to push the reset button so that your metabolism, your hormones, your inner workings can return to normal, allowing you to burn fat 24/7. With this approach, weight loss isn't something you accomplish through tiny, tasteless meals and draining workouts, but through an entirely new lifestyle you'll adopt one day at a time. The end result? A body that is constantly burning fat, no matter what you're doing, while you enjoy the process.

Adam did it, and now he has an entirely new life. You can, too.

If you've tried all the diets and are still struggling to lose weight, then you'll find this book very refreshing. Most diets focus only on dietary changes, and that's why their success is short lived. In contrast, *The All-Day Fat-Burning Diet*'s unique approach to weight loss is so effective because it harnesses the combined power of clean eating, smart exercise, and optimal rest and recovery. It helps you reestablish a healthy relationship with food and provides a flexible dietary and exercise framework that can be enjoyed for life.

You are about to experience the only dietary plan that resets your metabolism to lose up to 5 pounds per week using a unique 5-day food cycle that mirrors and honors your body's natural rhythms. And you'll do it without calorie counting, dogmatic diet rules, or long hours of exercise. Plus, the foods you'll eat will be delicious. I hope you're excited. I certainly am.

Let's begin.

# Part I

# Why Your Body's Not Letting You Lose Weight

# CHAPTER 1

# IS YOUR BODY STOPPING YOU FROM LOSING WEIGHT?

I'd like you to do something for me: Dust off an old photo album that contains those treasured photos of your parents when they were young. Flip through those pages, paying particular attention to any photos of large family gatherings. Notice anything? (Aside from the retro fashions, that is.) If you can't get your hands on an old family album, just do a Google search for group photos from the 1960s or even earlier. Anything jump out at you?

If you look around today, whether while walking down the street or watching one of the many reality shows on TV, I guarantee that you'll see a much different picture. If you take public transit or live in a big city, you have plenty of opportunities to spot what I'm talking about: Most people nowadays are so much heavier than people were 50 years ago! They are easily 20 to 30 pounds heavier, on average. It's not an exaggeration, no matter how much I wish it was. The proof is literally frozen in time for everyone to see.

Faded photographs aside, figures back up this observation. In the 1960s, the average American man between the ages of 40 and 45 weighed 169 pounds. By the year 2000, that average weight was 196 pounds![1] According to 2012 stats from the *Journal of the American Medical Association*, 16.9 percent of 2- to 19-year-olds and 34.9 percent of the 78.6 million American adults who were 20 years or older were obese.[2] What's scary is that those numbers didn't even include another 35 percent or so of adults who didn't qualify as obese but were still overweight and also at risk of weight-related problems like heart disease, stroke, type 2 diabetes, and certain types of cancer. And this isn't just happening in North America, either.

On a recent trip to Barbados, I decided to take a tour of the island. (It took a whopping 2 hours, as it's less than half the size of New York City.) During the excursion, the tour guide mentioned that even though this tiny Caribbean island was sheltered from the weight-gain epidemic for most of its existence, everything changed about 20 years ago. He revealed weight-gain numbers almost identical to the ones I mentioned above. What's going on? What changed? What's happening in our modern world that's making people around the globe—even on distant islands—so much heavier?

## YOU'VE BEEN LIED TO

For years, you've been told that losing weight is simply a matter of moving more and eating less. It's a simple formula that everyone can recite, with the net difference between calories consumed and calories burned being the name of the game. As such, if you've had trouble losing weight—as so many of us have—the thinking is that you simply need to work harder and be more disciplined. If despite your best efforts you still weren't able to lose weight, the judgment is typically that you lack willpower—you're lazy! Sadly, amid the stares of disapproval and humiliating, unasked-for opinions about your weight, you're probably judging yourself more than anyone else is. It's all your fault.

I'm here to tell you that's nonsense.

On a very basic level, calories do matter, but they pale in comparison to what your body is dealing with every second of every day without you even realizing it. As you go about your daily life, little do you know that underlying, invisible forces are likely stopping you from losing weight, holding you back, and making you miserable. Invisible forces? What are these invisible forces?

These nefarious, unseen forces are anything that puts your body out of balance, a precious state of optimal function known as *homeostasis*. These culprits are things we regularly contend with without giving them much thought: toxins, chronic stress, sugar (specifically, fructose) overload, and insufficient and/or poor-quality sleep.

Combine these culprits with misinformation about how and what we should eat—given to us by medical authorities who really should know better—and it becomes all too confusing. These factors create a lethal cocktail that affects every cell, organ, gland, and major system in your body. With their unrelenting presence wearing you down day after weary day, they eventually lead to increased inflammation, disrupted hormone levels, and a toxic overload in your cells and organs. All of this causes you to store fat. This dangerous tango with homeostasis is not to be taken lightly. Your body perceives any chronic influence that affects this ideal state as nothing less than a threat to your survival. When that happens, your body gradually shifts from thriving mode to surviving mode.

Unfortunately, these health disruptors are part and parcel of a modern life that our bodies were not designed to deal with. No matter how fast the world around us speeds up, we're still tackling it with the same factory-installed settings we inherited from our ancient ancestors. For example, life might be a lot more manageable if we could go for weeks without sleeping, but we haven't evolved that capability. Epigenetics, the science of how our environment and genes interact, is starting to reveal that the world we've built has been taking a toll on us at a genetic level that makes our weight and health problems even worse. Under the pressure and strain of modern living, we experience two key, undesirable side effects.

**FAT STORAGE INCREASES.** Since your body is under constant threat, your adrenal glands pump out cortisol, which flicks the switch to store more fat. Our biology is such that fat storage is an energy preservation mechanism in times of prolonged stress.

**SEX DRIVE PLUMMETS.** Since survival is the highest priority, reproduction takes a seat on the bench. If your body is constantly stressed, its main objective is to ensure your immediate survival, not that of your future offspring. And since increasing cortisol literally shuts off testosterone, it becomes more difficult to burn fat and maintain lean muscle.

In the terrific book *The Adrenal Reset Diet* by my close friend—and possibly the smartest man on the planet—Alan Christianson, NMD, there's a clear outline of the link between chronic stressors and fat storage. Note that "stress" is much more than just worrying about stuff. It's toxic overload, low blood sugar levels, excessive exercise, poor sleep, and pretty much anything else that offsets your body's desired state of balance (homeostasis), thus triggering its survival mode.

Dr. Christianson explains that our adrenal hormones control a switch that sends calories to our belly fat or to our muscles. When this switch is set to "fat storage," calories are sent to your fat cells. When the switch is set to "energy creation," these calories are sent to your muscles to be used as fuel. What makes this switch flip either way? When we perceive danger or any kind of threat to our well-being, even if it's simply a stern lecture from a boss or a lover, our "fight-or-flight" response kicks in immediately to help us fight or run away. Thus, our muscles require large amounts of quick energy to perform either task.

But during this acute bout of stress or danger, our muscles cannot burn and store energy at the same time, so calories are diverted to our visceral fat (the fat around our vital organs—belly fat) to be stored. Normally, animals—including us—can control their body weights quite effectively within a certain range. In response to stress, the adrenal glands release cortisol into the bloodstream, and how that cortisol acts depends on whether we're in surviving or thriving mode. When we're chronically stressed (survival mode), the cortisol causes us to slow down and store fat. When we are thriving, we eat in response to hunger, can use this food for energy, and maintain a healthy weight.

Short-term stress does not create weight gain until there is a disruption in this adrenal rhythm. Recall that since the beginning of the human species, our bodies have learned that bad things don't happen during times of plenty, only during famine or imminent danger. To survive and propagate the species, we simply stored fat. If we couldn't, we would have perished.

## WHAT'S HALTING YOUR FAT LOSS

Don't be surprised if this discussion is already setting off some alarm bells for you. Chronic stress, which puts your body into survival mode, is probably a big reason why you're dealing with unexplained weight problems. When was the last time you were without a care in the world?

Now, let's dig a little deeper and uncover some of the fat triggers that make matters worse. In the next chapter, we'll look at the six primary hormones and bodily functions that these fat triggers disrupt, making weight gain and fat storage almost unavoidable. But the good news is that when we address each of the fat triggers I'm about to discuss, the six big problems begin to resolve. To have better fruit, you must start at the root. That's what we're doing here.

Please note that I haven't included stress in this list because, in reality, chronic stress is the *result* of these issues. As you neutralize them by following the 5-Day Food-Cycling Formula outlined in this book, your body will switch from its stressed-out, fat-storing survival mode to thriving mode and you will become a healthier, leaner, fat-burning machine. Sound good?

### FAT TRIGGER #1:
### *Allergenic Foods That Cause Inflammation*

Have you ever been told to avoid eating gluten or dairy products? That's certainly a recommendation I've made for years to my clients and online audience. The reason is that these foods trigger inflammatory responses in your body that make losing weight and enjoying good health almost impossible. Not everyone is sensitive to them and not everyone will respond in exactly the same fashion, but I have yet to work with a human being on this planet whose health and waistline have not improved as a result of avoiding (or at least minimizing) these allergenic foods.

Let's look at each one more closely to see how it causes your body to hold on to fat.

## Wheat (Gluten)

You've certainly heard a great deal of terrible things about gluten in recent years. It's become the villain of the day with the alternative health crowd, and the witch hunt for the stuff has even made it into the mainstream. There seems to be a gluten-free option for everything these days. So, two questions you might naturally have are, What is it exactly, and is it really that bad for you?

To answer the first question, gluten is a protein composite (gliadin and glutenin) found in wheat, barley, and rye. It gives elasticity to dough, helping it rise and keep its shape, and often gives the final baked product a chewy texture. It's kind of like glue, hence the name. As for the second question, the answer is simple: Yes, it's really that bad for you.

There's a good reason why gluten-free products have become perhaps the hottest trend in food right now: Wheat products are some of the greatest contributors to obesity, diabetes, heart disease, cancer, dementia, depression, and so many other health problems. Who knew all of these problems could be caused by something as simple as a diet consisting of bread, cereal, and pasta? Having had those foods as the staple of my diet for nearly 20 years, I can attest to the sneaky health-robbing powers they possess. My personal beef with gluten is based on years' worth of research as well as my own personal suffering; since wheat consumption has been shown to cause celiac-like inflammation of the skin and hair follicles,[3] it's no surprise that it was one of the major factors in my developing alopecia.

I know it's hard to believe that wheat could wreak so much havoc on your health, especially when it's touted as such an important staple of a healthy diet. However, you have to bear in mind that this is not the same wheat that your grandparents were eating. What you eat today is drastically modified "Frankenwheat."

For this, you can "thank" Norman Borlaug—often referred to as "the

Man Who Saved a Billion Lives."[4] Borlaug was perhaps the most noted agronomist of the 20th century, and his effort in the 1960s to increase the global yield of wheat through hybridization techniques was born of noble intentions: His goal was to feed the drastically increasing numbers of starving people in the developing world. The resulting semidwarf, high-yield, disease-resistant wheat strain fulfilled his mission and won him a Nobel Prize, but his invention has inadvertently made millions of people sick and fat. Modifications have continued over the past 50 years, using techniques that include hybridization and chemical, gamma-ray, and x-ray mutagenesis. The latter has been used to develop a new "superstrain" of wheat, called Clearfield, that is herbicide resistant. These modern, mutant strains of wheat are a far cry from the wheat spoken of in any holy book.

You would think that the litany of studies showing the health issues related to these modern wheat strains would spur a return to older varieties, but this hasn't been the case. A big part of the problem is that massive money and power support big grain lobby groups like the Grain Foods Foundation and the Whole Grains Council. For decades, these groups have brainwashed us into believing that whole grains should be an essential part of our diets and that the fiber in their breads and cereals is good for lowering our cholesterol and improving other health markers.

There's a theme here that comes up time and time again when digging into the dirty laundry of the modern diet: When we start playing around with Mother Nature, we end up with far less predictable and less controllable outcomes. It's kind of like *Jurassic Park*.

As of 2014, the average American consumed about 179 pounds of wheat every year.[5] That's the weight of an entire person! Let's now look at how this engineered wheat affects our bodies.

- It contains amylopectin A–the most quickly digested and fattening form of starch.
- It contains a form of gluten that is superinflammatory.
- It is highly addictive, which makes you crave and eat more of it.

**Amylopectin A**

Amylopectin A is a superstarch found in modern wheat that makes our bread nice and fluffy. However, it's also a big part of the reason why a single slice of whole wheat bread (yes, even more so than white bread) now raises your blood sugar more than if you had consumed 1 table-spoon of table sugar![6] As you'll discover throughout this book, the higher the blood sugar response after consumption of food, the greater the release of your fat-storing hormone—insulin—and the more fat that can potentially be stored in your body. By contrast, beans and legumes contain amylopectin C—the least digestible form of the starch—which actually ends up feeding the good bacteria in your gut, making its sugar less available for absorption. As a result, it doesn't cause a spike in your blood sugar.

As if that wasn't enough, amylopectin A not only spikes our blood sugar more viciously than do other starches, it also leads to the develop-ment of insulin resistance. In fact, a study in the *Journal of Nutrition* showed that it actually causes nonreversible insulin resistance in rats.[7] It's helpful to understand that insulin resistance can be reversed through diet and exercise alone in most cases. However, this study showed that was impossible after just 16 weeks on a high–amylopectin A diet.

Wheat consumption stimulates insulin-mediated fat storage, which is mostly directed to visceral fat—the fat around the organs in your gut. The bigger your belly gets, the poorer your response to insulin becomes because the deeper layers of visceral fat are less responsive to it. They ultimately demand more insulin, which eventually leads to insulin resistance, or diabetes.

**How Gluten Causes Inflammation**

When you think of inflammation, you might think of the swelling you see when you mistakenly hit your thumb with a hammer. As painful and frustrating as that may be, it's a healing mechanism your body has in place to help heal the injury. What you might not realize is that inflammation happens inside the body as well, where you can't see it. When this hidden inflammation is ongoing, it can lead to all kinds of health problems. Can you imagine your whole body swelling up on the inside? It's an unpleasant thought, and the scary reality is that many of us live day to day like this without knowing it.

Plenty of things give rise to this situation, and gluten is one of them. Gluten creates a cascade of low-level inflammation reactions throughout your body that, over time, can lead to a host of bigger problems. At the highest level, gluten can lead to full-blown celiac disease—an autoimmune disease that triggers body-wide inflammation leading to insulin resistance, which causes weight gain, diabetes, and more problems.

Celiac disease results when the body creates antibodies against gluten that attack the lining of the small intestines, the main absorptive area in your body, which also provides a barrier separating you from your poop. This can lead to cramping, diarrhea, yellow stool, or even no symptoms at all in many cases. Over time, the destruction of the intestinal lining diminishes the amount of nutrients you can absorb from your food, leading to many nutritional deficiencies.

The protein in wheat, gliadin, has been shown to trigger the release of a protein called zonulin, an important gatekeeper of intestinal permeability.[8] The more wheat you eat, the more zonulin you activate, and the weaker the tight junctions become in your small intestines. This broken-down intestinal lining then allows the protein components of wheat (and other food proteins) to seep into the bloodstream, where a range of nasty immune and inflammatory responses begins.

But there is another kind of gluten sensitivity that results from a generalized hyperactivated immune system. This means that you can be sensitive to gluten without having full-blown celiac disease and still have inflammation and many other symptoms. On top of all this, a nongluten glycoprotein in wheat called wheat germ agglutinin (WGA), found in highest concentrations in whole wheat, increases whole-body inflammation. And whole-body (or systemic) inflammation is strongly related to heart disease and cancer.

A study in the *Journal of the American Medical Association* revealed that hidden gluten sensitivity (elevated antibodies without full-blown celiac disease) was shown to increase risk of death by 35 to 75 percent, mostly by causing heart disease and cancer.[9] Remember, gluten can trigger these same problems even if you don't have full-blown celiac disease. Many people have elevated antibodies to gluten without even knowing it. The best course of action is to simply assume you do, too, so that you avoid the deleterious effects of gluten.

And a word of caution: Don't be fooled by all those boxed and packaged "gluten-free" products you see scattered throughout the grocery store. Many of them simply replace gluten with other unhealthy, fattening ingredients like cornstarch, palm oil, and sugar. Don't fall for the manufacturers' sneaky tricks or eat too many of the foods I call gluten-free junk food, such as gluten-free cookies, cakes, and processed food. Processed food has a high glycemic load. Just because it is gluten-free doesn't mean it is healthy. Gluten-free cakes and cookies are still cakes and cookies! Vegetables, fruits, beans, nuts and seeds, and lean animal protein are all gluten free—stick with those.

## Gluten Addiction

It's hard to eat just one doughnut, isn't it? I'll be very honest with you—pizza is my nemesis, and I know why. At some level, I'm addicted to it, and that's likely because I've eaten tons of it over the course of my life. I certainly don't eat much of it now, but I scarfed so much of it in my childhood that a deep craving for it has probably embedded itself inside me. Even now, it returns from time to time, especially in moments of stress when my body just needs a comforting "fix."

Wheat's addictive properties are largely due to the fact that, upon digestion, its proteins are converted into shorter opioid-like proteins called gluten exorphins or gluteomorphins. They act in similar fashion to the endorphins you get from a runner's high by binding to the opioid receptors in the brain. That process is also responsible for the high you get after taking an illegal drug, setting the stage for an addiction similar to but probably less intense than heroin addiction.

Every now and then I get an intense craving, and when that happens, I'll bake myself a gluten-free pizza. I make a damn good pizza, but even that doesn't completely satisfy me. Even with all the fixings, that pie simply doesn't fool the reward center in my brain, which swiftly issues a gnawing craving, egging me on to get the real deal. Thankfully, I've become aware of these patterns, which makes it easier to put a stop to them when they arise. You can learn how to do the same thing by reading this book.

I hope by now you have a much better understanding of why wheat is terrible for your health and your ability to lose weight. It has no redeeming qualities, no matter what any dietitian, the American Diabetes Association, or even the latest food pyramid may tell you. Some of these authorities will likely tell you that if you don't have the HLA-DQ gene or specific antibodies against gluten, you'll be fine eating copious amounts of bread. I'm here to tell you otherwise. Let me save you the hassle of going through all sorts of blood and genetic tests. Let's just agree that wheat is not good for your body, okay? For that reason, none of the recipes in this plan—or any others that I ever create—will contain wheat or gluten. You don't need it, and you certainly won't miss it when you're enjoying delicious meals that help you drop a few pounds in the space of a few days.

## Dairy

I don't often speak poorly of others, and I don't consider myself a conspiracy theorist. However, when it comes to dairy, I consider it my duty to let you know about some pretty shocking schemes that have led you to believe that milk is not only necessary for good health, but also helps you lose weight.

Before I blow the whistle, let me first tell you why, despite some suspicious research and misleading ads, cow's milk really doesn't do a body good. The trouble with cow's milk (and its cheese and yogurt by-products) is the inflammation that it causes inside our bodies as a result of the proteins it contains, such as casein. Additionally, many people are lactose intolerant, which means they lack the enzyme *lactase* that digests the lactose sugar molecule. This can lead to many gastrointestinal symptoms like cramping, gas, diarrhea, and more.

If your gut is compromised, you're even worse off. If you have compromised intestinal permeability, or "leaky gut," it's more likely that your immune system will respond to potentially allergenic components in milk such as alpha- and beta-casein, casomorphin, and butyrophilin. This is especially true for people who are gluten intolerant, because it has been shown that milk proteins commonly cross-react with gluten. To put it another way, if you react to gluten, it's more likely that you'll also react to milk.

The other reason I discourage dairy consumption is that I personally think it's quite odd that we feel the need to drink another animal's milk to meet our protein and calcium needs. We're the only species on the planet that does this. Obviously, other animals don't have the means to milk another animal, but I'd be surprised if they would even if they had the capability of doing so.

As I discussed in *The All-Day Energy Diet*, the main issue with dairy is that it's the most acid forming of all foods. Considering that too much acid in our bodies—a condition known as *metabolic acidosis*—has been shown, like inflammation, to be at the root of many health problems we now face, it's a smart idea to minimize your intake of such foods. What's the problem with too much acid, and how does it make losing weight more difficult, you ask? When you eat any food, it is eventually metabolized by your kidneys, where it leaves either an acid or alkaline "ash." With continued consumption of acid-forming foods (dairy, grains, sugar, lots of animal products), we develop low-level acidosis, which must be buffered at the expense of alkaline reserves like bicarbonate and calcium.

Instead of allowing excess acid to ruin your delicate blood vessels and organs, your body looks to store this acid to prevent further damage. And guess where it goes? That's right—into your fat cells. Foods that contain more protein and phosphorus and fewer alkaline minerals like magnesium, calcium, and potassium are more acid forming, while those that have the opposite makeup are alkaline forming. Dairy products (especially cheese) are the most acid forming of all foods. This is due to the large amount of protein and phosphorus they contain. Even though dairy also contains a substantial amount of calcium, its phosphorus impairs calcium absorption and utilization in the body.

When you look at bigger, unbiased studies, dairy's true colors are revealed. Take, for instance, the Harvard Nurses' Health Study, which included more than 77,000 women. It found that women who drank three or more glasses of milk a day had no reduced risk of hip or arm fractures during a 12-year follow-up period when compared with women who drank little or no milk.[10] Or consider a large review in the journal *Osteoporosis International* involving a total of 39,563 men and women. It revealed that people who consumed less than one glass of milk a day were at no greater risk of bone fracture.[11] And many studies show similar results.

What's interesting is that our Paleolithic ancestors didn't drink milk, and yet osteoporosis was almost nonexistent in their time. Instead, they got plenty of natural sunlight, regular weight-bearing exercise, and lots of whole foods—the perfect recipe for strong bones. Yet, today, we continue to be misled by big-money lobby groups who want us to believe that milk is required for good bone health.

We've been duped, and it's all thanks to efforts like the $200 million campaign several years ago claiming that drinking milk was helpful for weight loss. You have to wonder where that conclusion came from, as a review of 41 randomized clinical trials, including a Harvard Medical School study, demonstrated that milk did nothing of the sort. The review asserted that the idea "has been totally discredited by research not funded by the National Dairy Council (NDC)."[12] And yet, for some reason, the NDC was allowed to run ads for years that featured slogans like "Milk your diet. Lose weight!" and suggested that three daily servings of dairy products could contribute to weight loss. It wasn't entirely untrue. After all, the more milk you drank, the more money ended up in their pockets, leaving yours lighter.

You may recall their other ads, like the highly visible "Body by Milk" campaign, which was aimed at teenagers and featured celebrities such as baseball star Alex Rodriguez and *American Idol* winner Carrie Underwood. It was quickly followed by the Physicians Committee for Responsible Medicine asking the FDA to prevent packaged dairy products from claiming links between weight loss and dairy consumption. (That ad campaign, like many others, based its ludicrous claims of weight loss on a select number of tiny studies—involving fewer than 100 people!—conducted at the University of Tennessee by Dr. Michael

Zemel, who received $1.68 million in grants since 1998 from the NDC. How is that even possible?)

Eventually, thanks to increased pressure, very little proper science to back up these claims, a significant lawsuit, and a reprimand from the US Department of Agriculture, the milk industry abandoned their ridiculous campaigns.[13] They may have received a much-needed scolding, but the damage was already done. Millions of people still believe that dairy products are good for your bones and help you lose weight. To this day, you'll find ads claiming this. It boggles my mind. Given that dairy is such a common allergenic food that can lead to a host of digestive and inflammatory issues—all of which can make losing weight more difficult—you should avoid it on this program if you truly want great results.

## FAT TRIGGER #2:
### *A Sedentary Lifestyle and Exercise Extremism*

My kids love the movie *Wall-E*. Okay, I do, too. It's pretty awesome. If you've seen the movie, you'll undoubtedly remember the grossly overweight humans on the spaceship being transported around in what seem like floating wheelchairs. In the slothful future in which the movie is set, they had become so lazy that they no longer knew how to walk. They say the best comedy is born of tragedy, so maybe that's why it's so funny. If you ask me, we might not be too far from this ridiculous scenario if we continue on our current path.

It doesn't take a rocket scientist to realize that if we don't move enough, we won't be burning calories, and thus we will have trouble losing weight. In fact, we're much more likely to gain weight, especially if we continue eating higher amounts of the wrong foods. Check out these frightening statistics: According to a 2008 Vanderbilt University study of 6,300 people, it was estimated that the average American spends 55 percent of his or her waking hours (7.7 hours) sitting or sedentary.[14] A 2010 study by the American Cancer Society found that women and men who were inactive and sat for more than 6 hours a day were 94 percent and 48 percent more likely to die prematurely, respectively, than their counterparts who sat less than 3 hours a day.

We also have to take into consideration what happens inside our bodies when we're sitting down. Sitting decreases the activity of an enzyme called *lipoprotein lipase* (LPL), which helps burn fat.[15] Too much sedentary time decreases bone mineral density without increasing bone formation, which raises the risk of fracture. Furthermore, excess sitting increases blood pressure and decreases the diameter of your arteries, both of which make heart disease more likely.[16]

What's even crazier is that these findings were just as strong in people who exercised regularly![17, 18] In our modern world, we believe that we can go to the gym for an hour and wash away all of our sedentary sins, but it just doesn't work like that. If you work in an office, commute by car, and watch a few hours of TV each night, it's not hard to see how you could spend the vast majority of your waking life (up to 15 hours a day!) sitting on your butt. This is a far cry from the evolutionary norms for humans and has serious consequences for our health.

Seeing mind-boggling numbers like I just showed you is one of the reasons that I now use a standing desk for most of my work. In fact, it's just my regular IKEA desk with another box on top of it so that my computer is at eye level as I'm standing. I now spend at least half of my working day standing and only use my couch (just opposite my desk) as my temporary reprieve.

The evidence is quite clear: If you reduce the amount of time spent sitting, regardless of whether you exercise or not, you can reduce your risk of obesity and early mortality. If you did nothing more than just stand more throughout the day, your body would be primed to keep you lean and healthy. How, you ask? It's simple, really—standing tones muscles, improves posture, increases bloodflow, ramps up your metabolism, and burns extra calories. If you think about it, it makes sense.

When you sit, your heart becomes lazy and doesn't have to work as hard against gravity to move blood to your upper body as it would if you were standing. Similarly, since few muscles are required when sitting, these unused muscles can weaken and atrophy over time, similar to what astronauts experience when traveling in the zero-gravity environment of outer space.

In Chapter 6, I'll show you some simple and powerful ways to prevent these problems from occurring—without exercising more. In the meantime, here's a simple truth to never forget: If you don't use it, you lose it. This goes for your heart, your muscles, your brain, everything!

Conversely, if you abuse it, you'll also lose it. I like to say that sitting is the new smoking, but actually, the same can be said for too much exercise. Who would have thought? With all these facts about how harmful too much sitting can be, you might be motivated to rush out to the gym, but not so fast. While some exercise of the right kind is terrific, too much may also be a major reason why you're holding on to weight.

Your body is always going, going, going, and like anything that's constantly in motion, it's subject to regular wear and tear. That's why, even as a fitness coach, I don't advocate excessive exercise. Going to the gym 5 to 7 days a week and killing yourself for up to 2 hours at a time creates a time bomb inside of you just waiting to go off. It might produce results in the very short run, but that level of intense activity is impossible to sustain. That's precisely why pro athletes fizzle out by the time they're 35 years old: Their bodies get beaten up and bottom out. It's impossible to sustain decades of the intense daily exercise they put themselves through.

I played pro soccer until I was 24 and later worked with hundreds of high-level collegiate athletes. I've seen firsthand what too much exercise can do to the human body. I won't lie to you and tell you that too much exercise will make you fat, because it won't. What it will do, though, is slowly destroy your body and make you look and feel at least 10 years older than your actual age. I'll share more of those insights and smart exercise solutions with you in Chapter 6, where I reveal how to train smarter using my LIFT method. For now, just understand that too much exercise (a really subjective determination based on many factors) can lead to overtraining, which has harmful effects on cortisol levels, thyroid function, and the immune system.

Research has shown that the cellular damage that occurs during overtraining can lead to nonspecific, general activation of the immune system, including changes in natural killer cell activity and the increased activation of peripheral blood lymphocytes. This hyperactivity of the immune system following intense overtraining can possibly even contribute to the development of autoimmune conditions, chronic fatigue, weight loss, decreased appetite, hypothyroidism, and sleep changes.[19, 20] Remember, the poison is in the dose. Too little or too much exercise can be harmful. We're after just the right amount to turn you into a healthy, fat-burning machine. That's what you'll learn how to do in this book.

## FAT TRIGGER #3:
## *Toxins*

Toxins come in all shapes and all sizes—from pesticides to plastic by-products and everything in between. They are found in our foods, in the water we drink, in the air we breathe, and even within our homes. Some of these toxic compounds have been banned, but the damage has already been done as they continue to bioaccumulate in the food chain and pose long-term challenges to the farming soils throughout America.

Our bodies were not designed to process these substances. For a disturbing look at the chemicals that breach the boundaries of our bodies, check out the Centers for Disease Control and Prevention (CDC) National Report on Human Exposure to Environmental Chemicals. It's downright terrifying. Scientists at the CDC found that nearly every person they tested was host to a boatload of nasty chemicals. They found flame retardants stored in fatty tissue and bisphenol A, a hormone-like substance found in plastics, excreted in urine. Even babies are contaminated. The average newborn was shown to have 287 chemicals in her umbilical cord blood, 217 of which are neurotoxic—poisonous to nerves or nerve cells.[21, 22]

This is serious stuff. Worse yet, these chemicals have not only been building up in our environment and food supply, but they're also abundant inside of our homes. A study as far back as 1985 revealed that the levels of numerous airborne chemicals were 10 times greater inside the home than outdoors![23] What's the problem with these toxins and chemicals? Can they really harm you and, for the purposes of our conversation here, make you fat? The answer is yes and yes.

A 2008 study in the prestigious journal *Lancet* showed that environmental toxins indeed make you fat and cause diabetes.[24] Toxicity is also a key metabolic problem for the two-thirds of Americans who are overweight. These chemicals contribute to weight gain in various ways, including disruption of the hormone-signaling system that regulates your metabolism, damage to and accumulation in your fat tissue, and increased risk for poisoning during weight loss,[25] as these toxins are released back into the circulatory system once that fat starts disappearing.

You probably know that your thyroid gland (and its hormones, especially T3) controls every aspect of your metabolism and thus how your body uses energy (or burns calories). Well, it's been shown that toxins have an inverse relationship with thyroid hormone function, so as levels of toxins in the blood go up, levels of biologically active thyroid hormone, T3, go down.[26]

To make the toxin-fat connection simple, here's a synopsis of how it all goes down in your body (based on our current understanding): Toxins negatively impact gene signaling within your fat cells and induce new fat cells to form while simultaneously increasing inflammation. Then, since many of these newly formed fat cells are themselves damaged by the toxins, they become metabolically impotent, which means they are unable to make leptin (the hormone that tells your brain that you have enough calories).[27, 28]

These damaged fat cells can swell like balloons as they fill up with more fat and toxins, making them unable to efficiently perform their normal functions. This leads directly to increased risk for type 2 diabetes via suppression of the important fat cell hormone known as adiponectin,[29, 30, 31] which normally increases insulin sensitivity and reduces tissue inflammation. Considering their direct impact on thyroid function; fat cell number, size, and function; and type 2 diabetes, I'm sure you can see that ridding your body of toxins is imperative for successful weight loss and overall good health.

Inside *The All-Day Fat-Burning Diet,* you'll discover how to purge your body of toxins through food and exercise alone. As you do so and we reduce the amount that continues to come in, your body will inevitably reset itself back to its factory-installed fat-burning settings.

## FAT TRIGGER #4:
## *Deadly Belly Bugs*

Most people are not aware of this, but the contents of your entire digestive tube (from mouth to anus) are actually considered to be *outside* your body. Its role is to selectively absorb nutrients, while keeping out dangerous compounds. What passes through the intestinal/gut walls is then considered *inside* the body. The rest is normally expelled in the stool.

A healthy gut is critical for ensuring that this process runs smoothly and that your body stays in good health. Since the beginning of time, we have evolved with numerous microorganisms that live on and in us, surrounding us at all times. In fact, we have 10 times more bacteria in and around us than we do human cells. This microbiome is critical to our health. Without it, we'd be dead. Unfortunately, many people suffer with a host of health issues (including weight gain) because this microbiome is completely out of whack.

Let me explain: Your gut (or large intestine) is host to hundreds of different types of microorganisms—trillions, in total numbers. These microorganisms communicate with your immune system and help to keep you healthy. But things can quickly go wrong if the balance of these microorganisms shifts in the wrong direction. *Dysbiosis*—the imbalance of good to bad bacteria—is a far too common problem in today's excessively clean, sugar-laden, and antibiotic-happy world.

Antibiotics—I call them A bombs—wipe out all bacteria in their path. The problem is that the bad kind have a tendency to flourish afterward much more rapidly since they're left unchecked by the good bacteria. This can lead to a vicious cycle of lifelong bacterial-related illnesses and a severely compromised gut. When you combine over-medication with food choices—like sugar—that feed our bad bacteria, it's no surprise we're dealing with more health problems than before.

A big reason for my developing an autoimmune condition when I was 17 years old was that my gut was severely compromised from years of dietary and medication abuse. Because I had eaten the very foods known to harm the sensitive gut lining and feed bad bacteria, like gluten and sugar, respectively, it's no surprise that this happened to me.

When you look at the rampant increase of autoimmune disorders today, it's pretty simple to understand what's happening: We are eating foods that hurt our gut, which in turn makes our gut more permeable to larger food proteins, or leaky. These larger proteins, which should normally be further broken down before being absorbed, seep into our bloodstream, which triggers an inflammatory immune response. The body responds in this manner since it considers these proteins foreign and potentially dangerous, even if they're seemingly harmless foods.

With constant exposure, these proteins can eventually trick our immune system into attacking our own body because many (for instance, gliadin from wheat and casein from dairy) closely resemble the proteins of our very own tissues. This is known as molecular mimicry, and it's one of the leading causes of a host of health issues. Take, for instance, Hashimoto's disease—a type of autoimmune disease that accounts for 90 percent of hypothyroidism cases, in which constant consumption of gluten (specifically, the protein gliadin) can turn the immune response against the thyroid. It's all because the protein in gluten resembles our thyroid tissue. Gluten isn't the only cause, but it plays a big part.

But let's bring this back to the gut and how it might be setting your body up to store too much fat. One such way is via the generation of toxins called lipopolysaccharides (LPS) that arise as a result of bacterial imbalance within your gut. These toxins have been shown to stimulate the formation of new fat cells, thereby promoting weight gain.[32] In addition, these cause leptin resistance, which significantly impairs your brain's ability to respond to the "I'm full" signal you get after eating. Thus, you tend to eat more.

It's not just the toxins coming from bad bacteria that prove problematic. The composition of bacteria within your gut can also be a big factor that determines whether or not you're set to gain and hold on to weight. A 2010 study in the *British Journal of Nutrition* showed that among 50 women, reduced numbers of the bacteria *Bifidobacterium* and *Bacteroides* and increased numbers of *Staphylococcus*, Enterobacteriaceae, and *Escherichia coli* were detected in overweight compared with normal-weight women.[33] Obviously, certain bacteria are not as desirable as others.

The dietary approach you'll discover in this book will help foster the good bacteria and starve off many of the not-so-good ones so that you can enjoy better health and easier weight loss. The best part is that this will all happen as a strategic by-product of simply eating the healthy foods you'll enjoy on the All-Day Fat-Burning Diet.

## FAT TRIGGER #5:
## *Sugar Overload*

It's fitting to follow the section on gut health with a discussion of one of the foods that's playing a leading role in ruining it—sugar! If you're someone who has a sweet tooth, then you undoubtedly know how challenging it can be to kick those sugar cravings. Sugar is an addictive drug, and it lights up pleasure centers in the brain in a way similar to what happens when we take hard-core drugs like cocaine and heroin.

I believe that added sugar is the single worst ingredient in the modern diet, especially as it pertains to fat loss. Numerous studies show that eating excess amounts of added sugar can have harmful effects on metabolism, leading to insulin resistance, belly fat gain, high triglycerides, and increases in dangerous low-density lipoprotein (LDL) cholesterol.[34, 35] Sugar is fattening, partly because it doesn't get registered in the same way as other calories by the brain, making us eat more. Not surprisingly, studies show that people who eat the most sugar are at a high risk of future weight gain and obesity.[36] That's frightening since our average sugar consumption has skyrocketed in the past 75 years with the advent of glass bottling technology, refrigerated vending machines, and the use of high-fructose corn syrup as a cheaper sweetening option.

At a very basic level, sugar makes you fat because it's quickly broken down and its glucose component spikes your blood sugar. As a result, insulin is released to remove all that excess sugar from the blood, and it's stored in your muscles, liver, and fat cells. The important thing to note is that your muscles and liver can store only so much in the form of glycogen before a "spillover" occurs. This leads to any additional sugar or carbohydrate being stored as fat.

Insulin is not your friend if your goal is to lose fat. Since insulin is a storage hormone, elevated insulin levels force you into fat-storing mode. Conversely, when insulin levels are low, your body can start breaking down fat for fuel—if the conditions are right.

But the problem with sugar doesn't just stop there. Sugar is actually 50 percent glucose (the form of sugar we just discussed that your body actually uses to produce energy) and 50 percent fructose. The latter is arguably even more devastating to your health and waistline. For years, the medical and dietary community has mainly been concerned with the glycemic index (GI) of foods, which only accounts for the glucose-mediated rise in blood sugar after eating a specific food. The glycemic index typically ranges between 50 and 100, where 100 represents the standard, an equivalent amount of pure glucose.

Foods with carbohydrates that break down quickly during digestion and release glucose rapidly into the bloodstream tend to have a high GI; foods with carbohydrates that break down more slowly, releasing glucose more gradually into the bloodstream, tend to have a low GI. A lower glycemic index is ideal since it suggests slower rates of digestion and a muted insulin response. Carbohydrates with a low glycemic index include slow-burning foods like beans and legumes, whereas breads and cereals tend to have a much higher glycemic index. It's no surprise, then, that the latter are more heavily involved in the development of diabetes and obesity.

The trouble is that nowadays almost all fast foods are loaded with high-GI carbs. Just walk into your local Starbucks and look at all the food options in the display case. What do you see? Bagels, muffins, scones, and a host of pastries. These are all high–glycemic index carbs that spike your insulin, increase your fat storage, and take you on an up-and-down energy roller coaster.

Now back to fructose for a second, because this is really important to understand: With all the attention that the glycemic index has received, many people have forgotten (or are completely unaware) that fructose is potentially a bigger problem. After all, the GI does not account for the fructose content in foods. And since table sugar is

50/50 glucose and fructose, we're overlooking a big piece of the puzzle. The trouble with fructose is that it cannot be used by our cells. It must first be metabolized by the liver and converted into glucose before it can be shipped to the rest of our cells to be of any use to us.

But here's the problem—our liver can process only so much fructose at once. It is a rate-dependent process, where any excess ends up being converted into uric acid and triglycerides. Think of it as an assembly line where parts move down the conveyor belt as workers deal with them in a timely fashion. Now, what would happen if the speed of the conveyor belt increased? Obviously, the workers would not be able to keep up and parts would be flying off the belt and piling up on the floor. That's what happens in your liver when you consume too much fructose. And here's the worst part—it doesn't take a lot of fructose to create this problem. Drink a can of soda or a bottled juice, and you're already there.

The only ways to avoid this backup and spillover into triglyceride formation are to eat less fructose (ideal), slow your intake of it, or exercise intensely (which is the only known way to increase your liver's ability to handle more fructose at once).

Understanding this is very important, especially if you're a relatively sedentary person. If you train like a pro athlete, then you have some more wiggle room, but the average person simply doesn't.

So fructose is bad news. Here are just a few more reasons why.

- Fructose forces your liver to create fats, which are exported as very-low-density-lipoprotein (VLDL) cholesterol (the most dangerous kind), leading to dangerous blood tryglicerides and cholesterol levels, fat around your vital organs, and, ultimately, heart disease.[37]
- Fructose increases blood levels of uric acid, leading to gout and elevated blood pressure.[38]
- It causes a buildup of fat in the liver, potentially leading to nonalcoholic fatty liver disease.[39]
- It causes insulin resistance, which ultimately leads to obesity and type 2 diabetes.[40]

- Fructose doesn't tell your brain that you're full, making you eat more total calories.[41]

- Excess fructose consumption may cause leptin resistance, throwing body fat regulation out of whack and contributing to obesity.[42]

When I talk about fructose, the most common question that arises is whether fruit, which contains fructose, is bad for us. The short answer is no. Fruits aren't just watery bags of fructose; they are real foods with a low energy density and lots of fiber. That fiber slows the release of fructose from the stomach into the liver. Since fructose metabolism is a rate-dependent process, the natural fiber found in fruit is the key. Knowing this will help you understand why eating an apple is much better for you than drinking apple juice. In fact, did you know that, ounce for ounce, apple juice and Coca-Cola have the exact same amount of sugar? Yup, 0.11 gram of sugar per milliliter. Crazy, right?

If you've followed my work, you'll know that I'm a huge proponent of juicing. But I'm not talking about juicing fruit. Why? Because when you juice fruit, you remove the fiber and create liquid fructose, which—although it may contain some good vitamins and minerals—is a health disaster in the making. If you're going to juice, and you totally should, focus on juicing vegetables. You can add in one apple or a pear for a touch of sweetness. But please don't juice five apples or two melons, okay? You're just asking for trouble.

So, to recap, eating fruit in its whole form is fine. Juicing it is not. And that holds true for those bottled, so-called healthy juices you find at Starbucks or your local grocery store. Look at their labels, and you'll see that they contain a truckload of sugar. Look at their ingredient list and you'll see why. Take Odwalla's Original Superfood Fruit Smoothie Blend as an example. Although it's cleverly disguised as a healthy green smoothie, it really isn't. Its ingredient list looks like this:

**Apple Juice, Peach Purée, Mango Purée, Strawberry Purée, Banana Purée, Spirulina, Soy Lecithin, Vitamin C (Ascorbic Acid), Kale, Wheat Grass, Barley Grass, Wheat Sprouts, Jerusalem Artichoke, and Nova Scotia Dulse.**[43]

And it contains soy! A green smoothie whose first five and thus more prominent ingredients are fruit juices and fruit purées? That's not much of a green smoothie, if you ask me. It's really a 450-milliliter dose of 49 grams of liquid sugar (more than in Coca-Cola), with just 2 grams of fiber. That's certainly much less fiber than you would get if you made a blended smoothie at home.

If you made a predominantly fruit-based smoothie (in a blender, not a juicer) at home, you would get a lot more fiber. Let me illustrate by showing you one of my favorite (although higher-carb) green smoothies. In it, I put:

| | |
|---|---|
| 2 cups kale or spinach | 1 pear |
| ½ cup cilantro | Juice of ½ lime |
| 1 apple | 2–3 cups water |
| 1 banana | |

When I calculate the nutrient breakdown (using cronometer.com), I get the following amounts of sugar and fiber.

**Sugar = 50 grams (about 25 grams of fructose)**

**Fiber = 14 grams**

That's a much different story than the bottled juice smoothie. Yes, this smoothie is higher in sugar, but much of it is buffered by a good amount of fiber. That's the difference when you make things from scratch versus relying on sneaky food companies.

## FAT TRIGGER #6:
## *Too Much "Frankenfood"*

Throughout this book, I'm going to drill something into your head: For the most part, being fat is not your fault. However, it is your responsibility to change—never forget that. I hope that becomes particularly clear when you see the impact of this next section. It should be pretty evident that you need to cut yourself a little slack.

We humans have the same neurobiology as we did hundreds of

thousands of years ago, but we now live in a much different environment. This has led us to eat more food without even being aware of it. Much of the blame rests in the hands of criminal food companies that have been allowed to get away with food-engineering nonsense for far too long. These products are sometimes called Frankenfoods. And you're about to see how they're destroying your body and making or keeping you fat.

There are many causes of obesity, but one indisputable fact is that calorie consumption has increased dramatically over the past few decades.[44, 45] It's important to keep in mind that it is not some collective moral failure that has driven our increased calorie intake. Instead, since all behavior is driven by our underlying biology and its interaction with our environment, we have to consider how the changes in our food supply have altered the way our brains and hormones work. In other words, changes in our food supply have caused malfunctions in our bodies, which are designed to protect us from getting fat. This is a big reason for the increased calorie intake and weight gain, *not* a lack of willpower.

I want to show you exactly how this is happening, to give you a better understanding of why you have food cravings, why you can't seem to pass on dessert even though you're full, and why even the best of intentions is futile when the wrong foods are in your house. To make sense of all this, it's important to first understand that your brain ultimately drives all your food-related behavior. *All of it.*

Your brain is always collecting information from inside your body and from your external environment. It then integrates that information to select the appropriate internal (physiological) and external (behavioral) responses. When it comes to food, your brain is constantly juggling your internal energy status (do you have sufficient calories?) and environmental triggers to determine the most appropriate digestive/metabolic (physiological) and eating (behavioral) responses.

If your body is low on energy (fat stores, calories), your brain will prompt you to eat. Likewise, as you're about to learn, when you see a TV commercial with a mouthwatering burger (environmental trigger), that, too, can lead to a greater desire to eat, even in the absence of hunger.

Much of our ultimate behavior has to do with dopamine centers in the brain. Dopamine is a neurotransmitter intimately involved with rewards. When we do something or eat something pleasurable, dopamine centers in our brains like the ventral tegmental area and the substantia nigra light up like fireworks on the Fourth of July. These areas then send information to other areas of our brains that prompt us to take action to get more of that good feeling. It's the same mechanism that creates a drug addiction or triggers any other type of highly rewarding behavior. Dopamine is a very important driver of behavior.

For instance, a study in mice showed that dopamine-deficient mice were totally unable to execute any goal-oriented behaviors. They would not even drink or eat until dopamine was surgically injected back into their brains.[46] It's that powerful! Dopamine thus plays a big role in how we select certain behaviors and helps to explain why eating chocolate cake is much more appealing than eating a boiled potato. More on that in a minute.

To help understand why eating certain foods is more appealing than eating others, we have to understand that our bodies (our brains, really) favor calorie density, fat, sugar, starch, salt, free glutamate, and the absence of bitterness. These are known as innate preferences. They are built-in factory settings that help explain why even babies prefer sweet foods over bitter ones.

As we go through life and eat various foods along the way, we develop "learned preferences," which are sensory properties that have been repeatedly associated with innately preferred properties. For instance, if we grow up eating sugary cereal and the ingredients in that cereal (think sugar, food dyes, etc.) excite our dopamine centers, we will learn to want more of that food. We learn that this specific cereal makes us feel good, and so we want more of it. It's classical conditioning at work, just like the famous Pavlovian study on dogs where the ringing of a bell triggered salivation due to the previous association of that bell with the arrival of food.

From a very young age, we have trained ourselves to desire certain foods over others. We will go to great lengths to eat these foods and, in most cases, will have too much of them, which contributes to weight gain. And if you think about it, it kind of makes sense. Food-reward associations likely evolved to guide us to scarce calorie-dense, nontoxic foods in our ancestral environment. If our ancestors had access to pizza and hamburgers, they would most certainly have chosen those over broccoli.

Eating 100 calories of broccoli requires a lot of broccoli. Eating 100 calories of pizza requires just a few bites. It's a more efficient way of consuming calories, which thousands of years ago is what our bodies

## Michelle's Story

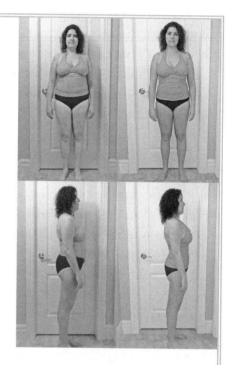

What Michelle went through on this program was nothing less than a transformation.

When she first started the All-Day Fat-Burning Diet, Michelle weighed 155 pounds, but the weight was just one of her troubles. She was suffering from regular bloating and acne and, what's worse, had trouble fitting into her clothes. She was so insecure about her stomach that she'd taken to wearing her shirts untucked in an effort to hide it. Miserable, she rarely found the energy or inspiration to cook much other than pasta or unhealthy, easy-to-prepare meals.

Michelle soldiered on, however, relishing the meals on this plan and committing herself to the workouts. The pounds melted off as the weeks passed, and soon, she started wear-ing her shirts tucked in again. Her hair was fuller and stronger, and her acne was gone. By the time she completed her third round of the 21-day program, she weighed 137 pounds—a weight loss of 18 pounds!

would have wanted to do to survive in a scarce caloric environment. But we no longer live in a scarce caloric environment.

As I mentioned earlier, our main motives for eating come from our internal energy status and our external environment. When we eat to satisfy our internal energy needs, we are eating in response to our body's hunger signals, which tell us that more calories (energy) are required. However, when we eat based on external environmental signals, we are eating for other reasons. Just browse the Web for pictures of chocolate molten lava cake and see how your body responds. If you're like me and you love chocolate, then your mouth is probably already watering just reading these words. That's dopamine at work once again. Those dopamine receptors are anticipating the potential reward—your eating the chocolate cake—which would flood them with dopamine and make you feel alive, at least temporarily.

As you probably know from experience, that urge then persists. It doesn't just vanish into thin air. This is why food advertisements are so powerful. Their external signals (juicy hamburgers, fresh pizza right out of the oven) trigger one or more of our primal senses, which then prompt us to seek out that food. We don't stand a chance.

The other reason we tend to eat higher amounts of man-made processed foods is because they provide a weaker "I'm full" signal to the brain. Normally, when you eat food, your stomach stretches, which sends a hormonal signal to your brain to stop eating. Furthermore, when food reaches your small intestine, a similar signal is sent via hormones like peptide YY3-36 and cholecystokinin to notify your brain that you're satiated.

But here's the thing: Satiety does not correspond to the calorie count of a food. It is mainly affected by the *quality* of the food, specifically by the presence (or lack) of certain macronutrients. Protein, fiber, carbohydrates, and fat (in that order) have the greatest satiating effect. Thus, a high-protein, high-fiber meal like salmon with lentils will keep you full longer than a high-carb, high-fat meal like pasta with cream sauce.

Food companies know these facts all too well and specifically engineer their foods to be higher in carbohydrates, fat, sugar, and salt and lower in fiber and protein so that your brain has no choice but to crave more of them. Furthermore, the more palatable a food, the more you have to eat to achieve satiety. That's why, if you've lived on man-made Frankenfoods for years, it becomes a lot harder to give up those foods.

Let's be honest about something—kale isn't nearly as palatable as an Oreo cookie. That's why we don't willingly eat as much kale and why we can easily polish off a box of cookies in no time. We eat more of what tastes good to us.[47] Processed foods have been designed to taste great and stimulate our brain's dopamine-releasing pleasure centers. It's that simple.

Want a simple formula for how to eat more (almost uncontrollably)? Eat foods that taste good and are high in calories, low in fiber, and low in protein. That sounds like most fast foods, if you ask me. This is why being fat is really not your fault. If you've relied on fast processed foods for much of your life (haven't we all?), then your brain has had a lot of exposure to these highly rewarding (yet fattening) foods. It recalls the taste and how good certain processed foods made you feel. And it will go to great lengths to get more of them in spite of your best attempts to eat well.

I'm not saying that eating healthy is a lost cause, because it certainly isn't. However, it's helpful to understand the forces at play and to cut yourself a little slack. Willpower can take you only so far. Consider the following stats at the heart of why we've gained so much weight in the past 50 years.

- We've greatly increased our consumption of inflammatory vegetable fats (canola, soy, corn oils), yet animal fat consumption has actually decreased.

- In 1822, the amount of sugar consumed was equivalent to drinking one can of soda every 5 days. Today, we consume that same amount every 7 hours![48]

- The cost of food has plummeted since the 1930s, from 25 percent to 10 percent of disposable income, which means we've been able to buy and eat more food. And now 43 percent of our food expenditure occurs away from home (i.e., in restaurants, via takeout), compared to just 13.4 percent back in 1929.[49]

- There's more food variety than ever before. In 1980, the average US supermarket carried 15,000 food products. By 2012, that number had soared to 43,000 food products, which means there are more ways to eat the very foods and ingredients that are making us fat and robbing our health.[50]

When you combine all of these factors with the fact that food companies now engineer their foods to please our most primal desires, it's no wonder more people are overweight and obese than ever before. Our neurobiology has remained the same, but our environment has changed dramatically. To make matters even worse, once obesity is established, overeating becomes a self-sustaining habit that is very hard to break.

Why? A big reason is the hormone leptin. Under normal circumstances, your body fat secretes leptin in proportion to its size. The more fat, the more leptin. This hormone then tells your brain's command center—the hypothalamus—to stop eating because enough energy (i.e., fat) is present.

When you lose weight, fat stores decline and leptin goes down. The hypothalamus then kicks in and prompts you to eat more (and decrease energy expenditure), fat cells grow, leptin goes up, and food intake and energy expenditure normalize. So you'd think that having more fat would be a good thing since it tells your brain to stop eating, right?

Sadly, that's not what happens. As with many other hormones, the more that is present and constantly knocking on the door of its receptor site, the greater the likelihood that you lose sensitivity to that hormone. Essentially, you stop responding to it. In this case, too much body fat leads to leptin resistance, which means that leptin's "I'm full" signal does not reach the brain and you end up eating more and more food.

Leptin resistance is also significantly associated with inflammation response in the hypothalamus. Research has shown that C-reactive protein (a marker of inflammation) binds to leptin and attenuates its physiological functions.[51] So, anything that creates inflammation in your body (think gluten, dairy, alcohol, rancid vegetable oils, etc.) can eventually disrupt leptin signaling in the brain, which means that you're more likely to eat more food than your body really needs. It's also well known that fructose consumption causes leptin resistance,[52] so put down that can of soda or sugary bottled juice!

As you can see, an arsenal of internal and external factors influences how much we eat. And it seems when we override our internal needs by continually giving in to external temptations, our internal regulation of food intake eventually becomes severely disrupted.

An altered internal physiology, along with the external presence of foods engineered to be extremely tasty—high in sugar, fat, and salt and low in satiety-inducing protein and fiber—explains why we're fatter than ever before. It's also part of the reason why we're more likely to eat cheesecake after a big meal, even though we're stuffed, than a boiled potato.

Even though you do your best to eat well, you're still at the mercy of your environment, which can have a powerful effect on your food choices. For instance:

1. **If a food costs less and takes little effort to prepare, we tend to eat more of it.** Food companies know this. It's part of their gospel. After all, would you be more likely to eat a piece of chocolate cake sitting right in front of you that costs nothing or to run to the store, buy the ingredients, and make it yourself? I think the answer is obvious. That's why having readily accessible, convenient foods in your house is a disaster waiting to happen. Food that is immediately accessible is more likely to be eaten than food that takes more effort to prepare.

2. **If we eat with lots of people, we tend to eat more.**[53] I'm a big fan of social gatherings where we share food with friends and loved ones. It's one of the joys of life. However, the research shows that when we eat with six or more people, we tend to eat 72 percent more calories. I think that's partly because we get lost in conversation and the social ambiance and become less mindful of what and how much we're eating.

3. **Stress can make us eat more.** In the short term, stress causes the hypothalamus to provide corticotropin-releasing hormone, which suppresses appetite. The brain also sends messages to your adrenal glands to pump out the hormone adrenaline, which triggers the body's

fight-or-flight response and temporarily puts eating on hold. But if stress persists, it's a different story. The adrenal glands release cortisol, and cortisol increases appetite. Sadly, it doesn't increase your appetite for healthy foods. As you likely know, when you're stressed, you seek out foods high in fat, sugar, or both, which seem to calm the brain by inhibiting further activity in the parts that produce and process stress and related emotions.

4. **Lack of or poor-quality sleep can make us eat more.**
Sleeping and eating are intricately related.[54] Animals subjected to total sleep deprivation for prolonged periods end up eating dramatically more food.[55] In humans, the effects of lack of sleep or poor-quality sleep are similar and could be a significant contributing factor to our weight-gain epidemic. In 1960, American adults slept an average of 8 to 8.9 hours per night, whereas in 2002, research conducted by the National Sleep Foundation indicated that the average duration had fallen to 6.9 to 7 hours.[56, 57]

Normally, sleep is facilitated by a rise in melatonin and a drop in cortisol as the sun begins to set and our environment gets darker. During sleep, we see a greater release of growth hormone (for building and repairing cells) and a decrease in adrenal stimulation. However, inadequate or poor-quality sleep disrupts all of these responses, more readily activating our stress-response pathways, which tell our bodies to hold on to fat.

Additionally, sleep loss alters the ability of our hunger hormones— leptin and ghrelin—to accurately signal caloric need to the brain, leading to excessive caloric intake when food is freely available.

I hope you're getting the message that not enough or poor-quality sleep has dramatic and unwanted effects on your body that compel you to eat more food and gain more weight. In Chapter 8, Sleep Your Way Thin, I'll show you the best strategies to help you sleep better.

## PULLING THE TRIGGER ON FAT

In this chapter, I've summed up the major fat triggers literally forcing your body to gain weight. Many are beyond your control, while others are directly influenced by your daily actions. The All-Day Fat-Burning Diet is designed to eliminate (or at least minimize) each of these triggers, while resetting your metabolism so that you can start burning fat 24/7.

The exciting thing is that no matter how far gone you think you might be, there's always hope. There's always a light at the end of the tunnel. It doesn't matter if you weigh 400 pounds or 160 pounds and just want to lose a few pounds, this program can help.

Before we jump into how this program works, let's quickly turn our attention to how the fat triggers in this chapter affect some of the important hormones responsible for fat loss. Seeing how these hormones impact your ability to lose weight will help you understand why I designed this program the way I did.

CHAPTER **2**

# 6 REASONS WHY YOU CAN'T SEEM TO LOSE WEIGHT

If you've ever pored over lifestyle magazines and diet books trying to find the secret to weight loss that actually works, you've probably realized that almost every method is merely a remix of some other fat-blasting technique. The same exercises and meal plans seem to pop up again every few years, only with different names.

It begs the question: If these basic moves and meals are all it takes to get lean, why are so many people still struggling to lose weight? Most importantly, why are you? Hopefully, the last chapter opened your eyes to the fat triggers that have derailed your valiant but ultimately futile efforts to lose weight for good. It's not just a matter of eating less and exercising more. External forces have shaped your body into what it is today. Now let's look further into the internal forces at play as well.

Just hearing the word *hormones* might make you giggle a bit, because they're often talked about in a sexual context. However, the truth is that these microscopic chemical messengers affect just about everything taking place inside you. Think of them as tiny software programs that direct your bodily processes—everything from your body temperature and mood to your metabolism, growth, and even sense of balance!

If you've tried unsuccessfully to lose weight in the past, then working out more and eating less is most likely not your answer. You will be better served by first addressing and correcting the underlying issue—your physiology. So let's take a look under the hood to get a better understanding of why your body holds on to excess weight. Later in this book, I've outlined some clear tools and strategies to help you correct those physiological imbalances, but first let's examine what's going awry inside you.

## THE INSULIN, BLOOD SUGAR, AND FAT CONNECTION

You've undoubtedly heard in the last few years that eating sugar can be bad for you, but you may not understand why. And what's the difference between the sugar in the food you eat and blood sugar, which is circulating in your body?

Here's what you need to know: Blood sugar, or blood glucose, is stored inside of you and is the body's preferred source of fuel. It's what our cells use to produce adenosine triphosphate (ATP), the ultimate form of energy in the body. How does it get there? It's derived from the sugar in the food we eat (mainly carbohydrates) and from stored glycogen within our muscles and liver.

As with everything in the human body, there's a meticulous process through which sugar in your food becomes blood sugar and ultimately the energy you need to do everything from lifting a pencil to running a marathon. The key to this process is insulin, the hormone responsible for shuttling sugar out of your blood and into your muscle, liver, and fat cells.

Eat too much sugar, and regular waves of insulin will try to ferry it out of your blood. With constant exposure, though, your cells can become desensitized to insulin. The consequence—too much sugar in the blood—is dire, and sometimes even deadly. *Insulin resistance* is why two-thirds of Americans are overweight and why 10 percent of the world's population goes on to develop type 2 diabetes. As if that weren't bad enough, too much sugar in the blood will ruin your arteries, nerves, and other precious tissues. It also increases triglycerides (fats) in the blood, raising your risk of heart disease.

In fat cells, insulin resistance will trigger an increased release of hormone-sensitive lipase (HSL), resulting in further breakdown of triglycerides (stored fat) into free fatty acids. These free fatty acids (FFAs) then move to the liver. Here, FFAs can either be converted to ATP energy in the mitochondria, converted back into triglycerides for storage, or even incorporated into dangerous very-low-density lipoprotein (VLDL) cholesterol particles.

But it gets worse because insulin resistance also activates many of the lipogenic (fat-forming) genes in your liver, meaning that more sugar and FFAs will be converted into fat, rather than burned as energy. Similarly, too much sugar in the blood causes enzyme processes in the liver to favor the conversion of excess sugar into fat. Simply put, you get even fatter.

On the other side of the coin is fluctuating or low blood sugar, known as *hypoglycemia*. Although you might not think this would be problematic, it can be just as detrimental to your weight-loss efforts. Before my wife, Amy (whose nickname is Yammy), and I learned about nutrition back in our early twenties, she used to turn into what I called the Yammy Monster if she didn't eat frequently enough. You know the "hangry" feeling of being hungry and angry? That's hypoglycemia at work. The unwanted hangry symptoms of low blood sugar circle back around to insulin, once again.

The trouble with blood sugar fluctuations is that the highs elicit insulin release, which immediately stimulates the production of inflammatory chemicals, which in turn cause an increase in cortisol. Remember, inflammation is a form of stress and cortisol is one of your body's stress responses. In fact, any form of stress will create the same response. And since cortisol's primary function is to increase blood sugar, a vicious cycle of low blood sugar, high blood sugar, insulin release, inflammation, and cortisol release is started. Stated otherwise, you could have a perfect diet and exercise regimen, but if you have elevated cortisol levels, you may still suffer from blood sugar issues. I sure did for most of my teens, thanks to my high-sugar diet.

Insulin also has a number of unwanted effects that impair your ability to lose weight. First, insulin creates undesirable hormonal shifts in both men and women. In men, it upregulates an enzyme called *aromatase*, which converts testosterone to estrogen. The opposite reaction occurs in women. This makes fat loss more difficult for both sexes. Second, increased insulin levels are known to elevate leptin, one of our important hunger hormones. And as with insulin, chronically elevated leptin levels can lead to "leptin resistance," whereby the brain no longer responds to leptin and thus never gets the signal that you are full and should stop eating. Third, insulin stimulates an inflammatory chemical called interleukin-6 (IL-6), which has a number of damaging effects inside the body including raising cortisol levels even further. Finally, insulin impairs your liver's ability to clear toxins and excess hormones from your body. As a result, these compounds linger in the body longer than they should and cause further damage. For instance, having too much estrogen circulating in your body is not ideal as it promotes cell growth (i.e., cancer) and is the biggest factor in increasing fat storage at the hips and thighs by upregulating alpha-adrenergic receptors in those areas.

If your goal is to reset your body to become a fat-burning machine, then you have to control both blood sugar and insulin. And that is simply not going to happen if you eat constantly throughout the day or rely on refined carbohydrates that spike your blood sugar. Recall that, in a fed state, insulin goes up. Conversely, in a fasted state, it goes down. If you're constantly in a fed state because you're eating every 2 to 3 hours, then is insulin ever getting a break? Not really. That's just one reason for the strategic 5-Day Food-Cycling Plan in this book. Your body doesn't need a constant infusion of food. You'll see why when we get to Chapter 5.

The takeaway? If you've been having a tough time losing weight, then fluctuating levels of insulin could be at play.

# THE STRESS, CORTISOL, AND FAT CONNECTION

I've mentioned that stress and its ensuing cortisol release are big contributors to gaining and holding on to excess weight. Remember, when your body perceives a threat (a stressor of any form), it usually responds by storing and saving fat for a rainy day. This goes back to our Paleolithic environment. It's the classic fight-or-flight response that helped our ancestors survive, but it doesn't serve us well in today's nonstop stressed-out world.

The major reason that stress impairs your ability to lose fat is because it prompts the adrenal glands to release cortisol, whose main role is to increase blood sugar levels during times of stress. Thus, chronically high cortisol will lead to high insulin levels (due to constant high blood sugar), which as we just learned leads to fat storage.

Too much cortisol also impairs your ability to lose fat through the following mechanisms.

- It decreases your body's ability to make and convert thyroid hormone into its active form, T3, which results in a slowed metabolism since your thyroid is the master metabolism gland.

- It impairs your brain's ability to communicate with leptin (the "I'm full" hormone), which means you don't get the message and end up eating more.

- It lowers your body's ability to use insulin at the cellular level, which increases your chances of developing diabetes.

- Like insulin, it lowers your liver's ability to detoxify excess hormones and toxins, which leads to further hormone imbalances that contribute to weight gain.

- It increases imbalances in your gut flora (known as *dysbiosis*) and can lead to leaky gut, allowing large food proteins to enter your bloodstream, which can lead to heightened immune and stress responses.

Those are just a few of cortisol's effects on fat loss. The health implications of too much cortisol (and too little, for that matter) are just as bad. It's important to repeat: Stress isn't just worrying about

# Sandy's Story

As an occupational therapist, Sandy is required to be fully present with her patients, guiding them through their difficulties to make their lives more fulfilling. However, that's pretty hard to do when you're barely sleeping at night.

"I used to feel lucky if I got 5 to 6 hours a night," says Sandy. "I'd try to catch up on the weekend, but it barely worked. I was tired all the time, and it was hard to keep up with work."

Determined to make a change, Sandy jumped into the All-Day Fat-Burning Plan with vigor. Immediately upon starting, she was taken with the ease and simplicity of the plan, a stark contrast to other diets she'd tried and to the demands of her job.

"It really was a no-brainer," she says. "I made sure I had all the groceries ahead of time, and they were all simple items—nothing too exotic. It wouldn't take me that long to prepare my meals. That was a big help. The exercise only took me 30 minutes in the morning three times a week, and altogether, the program made me lose my cravings for salty or sweet stuff. I was surprised how easy it all was."

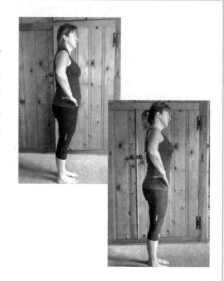

After a few weeks on this plan, Sandy dropped from 163 pounds to 152 pounds and went from a 33-inch to a 30-inch waist. It was exciting, she notes, but not as thrilling as the new sense of calm and restfulness in her life.

"I have a new energy, which is the most amazing thing. I was addicted to caffeine, but I'm happy to say I'm off of that now," says Sandy. "What's best of all is that I now get between 7 and 8½ hours of sleep a night. It's refreshing. I have more energy every day, and I stay focused in a way I couldn't before."

stuff. It's the foods you eat, how you exercise, the toxins you ingest, your mental and emotional concerns, and more. Anything that pushes your body out of balance (homeostasis) can be considered a form of stress. The goal of the All-Day Fat-Burning Diet is to minimize these stressors as much as possible by improving the quality of your diet, exercise, rest, and recovery.

Although the promise of this book is to help you lose up to 15 pounds in as little as 21 days following my proven 5-Day Food-Cycling Formula, the reality is that you can follow this way of eating and living forever. I do. It's not a fad. It's a principle-based program that resets your body to burn fat. I recommend following the plan for at least 21 days. Then you can continue to follow it to the letter or modify it slightly, as you'll see in Chapter 12, so you can stay lean and healthy for life.

## THE THYROID AND FAT CONNECTION

Stated simply, your thyroid is the gland responsible for your body's metabolic rate. Thus, anything that impairs its function will slow your ability to lose fat. Thyroid hormones, specifically the active form tri-iodothyronine (T3), act on nearly every cell in the body by increasing our basal metabolic rate and regulating pretty much all growth-related activity. These hormones also regulate protein, fat, and carbohydrate metabolism and stimulate vitamin metabolism.

How does the thyroid exert its powerful metabolic functions, and why does it help or impair your ability to lose fat? Well, a great deal of its power has to do with the fact that its hormones target the metabolic powerhouses inside our cells, called *mitochondria,* which are responsible for creating energy (ATP) and generating heat (as a by-product). Essentially, the more T3 reaching your cells, the more signals your mitochondria receive to produce energy (or burn calories, if you will).

The intimate link between mitochondrial and thyroid function is clear and can be seen in the changes that occur at the mitochondrial level with aging, exposure to cold, and feeding—three events also well known to greatly affect thyroid function.[1, 2, 3] Considering the thyroid's importance, it's sad to see that these days almost everyone has a thyroid condition. The thyroid is very sensitive to external chemicals like chlorine, lead, and mercury; to gluten and gut problems; and to low levels of important minerals like iodine and selenium. Thyroid toxins are prominent in our food supply and environment, so perhaps constant exposure to them has negatively impacted many people's thyroid glands.

Hypothyroidism (underactive thyroid) is more common in women than men and its prevalence increases with age (10 percent of adults over age 65 have it). According to a 2000 study, 1 percent to 2 percent of the US population has it.[4] Personally, I think those numbers are way too low. From what I've seen in my 2 decades of helping people get healthy and fit, I'd say 30 percent (or more) of the population has hypothyroidism.

## IS YOUR THYROID WORKING AGAINST YOU?

Here are a few more ways your thyroid impacts your ability to lose fat.

- Low thyroid function can arise from prolonged starvation. Thus, not eating, or restricting your calories for several days (or more), can hurt your thyroid and thus your ability to lose weight. This is why having a healthy feast day once a week can help you to lose weight.
- Low thyroid function affects important neurotransmitters in the brain (namely serotonin), resulting in sugar and fat cravings and overeating. Both contribute to weight gain.
- Low thyroid function decreases the production of growth hormone, a potent fat-burning hormone that is excreted especially during exercise and fasting states.

Cortisol, insulin, and toxicity (just to name a few) have a big impact on the complicated chain of events involving the thyroid, and that's why we aim to keep them in check in this program. As a result, you can feel good that you're doing your thyroid a much-needed favor and not creating an environment that taxes it further.

For instance, you can have subclinical hypothyroidism, meaning that a blood test would not detect any issue. However, monitoring your basal body temperature each morning for a week would tell you a much different story. Basically, a consistently lower-than-normal body temperature indicates that your thyroid is sluggish. If that's the case, you'll probably feel sluggish as well. In fact, how warm or cold you feel is an indicator of your body's metabolic function.

Symptoms of low thyroid include fatigue; sluggishness; fat gain; dry/brittle hair, skin, and nails; decreased motivation; forgetfulness; and cold hands and feet—just to name a few. The trouble with treating low thyroid is that many possible links in the chain can be broken, starting from the pituitary gland in your brain all the way down to the nucleus in each of your cells. Thus, it's not as simple as just taking more thyroid hormone.

For instance, you could have a pituitary defect (thank you, cortisol), which would impair the initial signal sent from your brain to produce more thyroid hormone. Or, if your liver is too toxic, it won't be able to convert inactive thyroid hormone, T4, into the active form, T3. Or there could be a problem with thyroid-binding globulin, which carries thyroid hormone around your body. There are many possible reasons for low thyroid symptoms, and that's why just ingesting more thyroid hormone may not always be the solution.

## THE GUT, IMMUNE SYSTEM, LIVER, AND FAT CONNECTION

As weird as it sounds, health (and thus fat loss) begins in the digestive tract, which includes the gut. In Chapter 1, we saw some eye-opening examples of how the modern gut, disrupted by environmental toxins, sugar, and antibiotics, has become a breeding ground for disease and fat gain.

Recall that an unhealthy gut is usually characterized by dysbiosis, or the imbalance of good to bad bacteria, which (in addition to allergenic foods like gluten) can promote the development of intestinal permeability (or "leaky gut").

A 2012 Brazilian study showed that intestinal permeability is a contributing factor to obesity.[5] The researchers in this study showed how two classes of foods—fructose and fat—play an important role in intestinal permeability and ensuing weight gain.

Fructose, they said, is thought to damage the liver directly by increasing blood levels of lipopolysaccharides (LPS), causing fatty liver, inflammation, and hepatic insulin resistance. All lead to weight gain and more serious health consequences.

Before we look at how to clean up your gut, let's look at how dysbiosis and leaky gut impact your ability to lose weight.

## Tina's Story

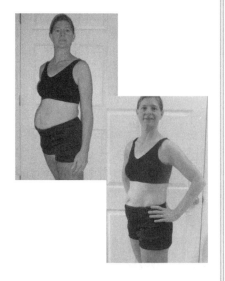

"I have stage 3 adrenal fatigue issues and have been on hydrocortisone, progesterone, testosterone, and Nature-Throid (for hypothyroidism) for months. I gave birth to the last of my 11 children more than 4 years ago. The last 2 years I have lost a good deal of weight, but over the past 6 months, I've been under lots of stress and have started gaining again.

"After just 7 days on the All-Day Fat-Burning Diet, the numbers were awesome! The length and timing (every other day) of the workouts makes them *so* doable. And the recipes . . . I feel that I have become a gourmet chef. Okay, maybe that is stretching it, but all the recipes are wonderful! Most days I'm not even hungry enough to eat three full meals, and I have so much energy that I forget to take my second dose of vitamins!

"After just a little more than a month, I've lost 4 inches from my waist and 2 inches from my hips. Thank you, Yuri!"

**THYROID DYSFUNCTION:** Approximately 20 percent of the hormone produced by the thyroid needs to be metabolized by gut bacteria to become active (the T3 form). However, dysbiosis decreases the amount converted, which then negatively affects your metabolic rate.

**INCREASED INFLAMMATION:** Leaky gut allows the entry of undigested food proteins and LPS into the blood, triggering systemic inflammation. As a refresher, inflammation primarily causes fat gain by triggering the stress response, which increases cortisol and initiates the cascade of consequences we discussed earlier.

**ESTROGEN OVERLOAD:** Dysbiosis can increase estrogen levels in the body by upregulating an enzyme called beta-glucuronidase, which severs an important connection in the liver responsible for removing estrogen from the body.

**NEW FAT CELLS:** LPS toxins from the gut have been shown to stimulate the creation of new fat cells, which then hold on to more toxins and fat.[6]

Think of your gut as the fortified walls around a castle. When the castle owner wants to allow people into the castle, he opens the large wooden door and those individuals may enter. Otherwise, enemies and dangers are kept at length by the impenetrable walls surrounding the castle.

Our bodies are built to function in the same way. However, years of dietary abuse, environmental toxins, and chronic stress have crumbled our gut walls. Now, instead of only the best nutrients being allowed to enter our bodies, we are invaded by unwanted food proteins and toxins that want to take over the castle. Most of us are walking around with compromised guts, and we're not even aware of it.

When anything (a nutrient, toxin, etc.) is absorbed *out* of your gut, it is sent to your liver for processing. It's very similar to what happens when you travel to a new country and must go through customs before stepping foot outside the airport. Your liver is your customs agent. However, while the nutrient or toxin is en route to the liver, if the immune cells around your gut lining perceive it as a threat of any kind, your body can start to mount an immune response and produce antibodies against that particular "invader." These antibodies are your body's defense troops.

But with constant exposure to the larger protein molecules that have been able to sneak past your compromised gut lining (thanks, leaky gut), your immune system starts to become hyperactive, almost like a paranoid mob boss looking over his shoulder every 2 seconds for the cops. A hyperactive immune system is not desirable since, in its confusion and increased sensitivity, it can start to confuse your own body tissue with foreign proteins. This is one way in which autoimmune disease, like Hashimoto's thyroiditis, develops. If your thyroid is compromised, you'll have a tough time losing weight. So let's keep your gut clean and keep those toxins at bay.

One of the best ways to accomplish these goals is to get rid of allergenic, inflammatory foods so that you give your gut and immune system time to settle down. That's just one reason why gluten and dairy are not part of the All-Day Fat-Burning Diet.

Remember, these hyperactive immune and inflammatory responses begin with what gets past your gut lining and the "customs agent" in your liver. The liver serves more than 500 functions in your body. One is detoxification—filtering and eliminating heavy metals, chemicals, toxins, excess hormones, cholesterol, bile, and anything else that will not serve your body. Detoxification is not a 10-day quick-fix process, but rather something that your body goes through 24/7, 365 days a year—forever! It's that important. It's as important as taking the trash out. (If you didn't, I'm sure you can imagine the nasty consequences of a few weeks, months, or even years of trash buildup in your house.)

Based on all the external reasons for fat gain discussed in Chapter 1, I think it's safe to say that we are all toxic. Pure and simple. More than ever before, we are exposed to hundreds of thousands of chemicals new to the planet and to the human species. Your goal is to reduce your exposure and keep your body as clean as possible, from the inside out. Otherwise, it breaks down and stores fat.

I've already covered how toxins from both internal and external sources have been shown to not just ruin our health but actually cause us to gain and hold on to weight. The good news is that by simply following the dietary and exercise recommendations in this program, you'll be doing your gut and liver a huge service. And you will feel and look better as a result.

## THE LEPTIN AND FAT CONNECTION

Leptin is one of your most important fat-loss friends because it's the main hormone that tells your brain when you're full. If leptin doesn't work properly, your brain doesn't get that message and you continue eating beyond your body's energy needs.

Leptin is made by adipose tissue (aka fat) and secreted into the blood, where it travels to the hypothalamus in your brain. Leptin tells the hypothalamus that you have enough fat, so you can eat less or stop eating. Generally, the more fat you have, the more leptin you make, and the less food you'll eat. Conversely, the less fat you have, the less leptin you have, and the hungrier you'll be. So, for weight loss, the more leptin, the better. Supposedly. But it isn't that simple.

After all, you would think that heavier people would somehow magically stop eating or start losing weight once their leptin levels were high enough. Unfortunately, as with insulin, you can become leptin resistant when too much leptin is bombarding your hypothalamus. Leptin resistance also occurs as a result of increased inflammation, which can alter leptin receptors in the hypothalamus. Fructose consumption is another culprit that severs the communication between leptin and the brain.[7]

So, you can have a lot of fat making a lot of leptin, but your brain might not be getting the message. Thus, it still thinks you need more food, and so there's no off switch. Regardless of how much you eat, your brain might think you're starving, because as far as it's concerned, there's not enough leptin. So it makes you even hungrier. It's a vicious cycle. Leptin also responds to short-term energy imbalance: A severe caloric deficit will result in reduced leptin secretion. This is your body's way of getting you to eat when you need energy. Likewise, temporary overfeeding boosts leptin, reducing hunger.

If you look at wild animals, they eat when they're hungry and stop when they're full. Obesity is extremely rare in the wild when animals eat their native diets. But normally, wild animals eat varying amounts of food, sometimes gorging, sometimes fasting. They never count calories, and yet these animals seem to be experts at maintaining excellent body composition. Obviously, something we humans are doing (or eating) isn't working.

Much of our knowledge of leptin comes from the study of two types of lab mice—the ob/ob mouse, deficient in genes responsible for leptin production, and the db/db mouse, deficient in the leptin receptor gene. The former responds to leptin but produces none, while the latter produces plenty but responds to none. An ob/ob mouse suffers from an uncontrolled appetite. It is literally always hungry and massively obese, because the normal satiety-signaling hormone—leptin—is absent from its body. However, when you inject an obese ob/ob mouse with leptin, it loses weight and its health markers normalize. Its appetite dwindles to normal, and its energy balance is restored.

But when you inject an obese db/db mouse with leptin, it doesn't improve. It already has high circulating leptin, since its considerable fat stores are secreting it, but there is no receptor to accept it. This gives us important insights into the power of leptin and its receptors in the hypothalamus. How do you restore healthy leptin communication so that your body actually knows when you have enough energy and can stop eating?

The answer is simple in theory but perhaps tougher in practice. Much as with insulin resistance, the key is reducing inflammation in the body and avoiding the foods that cause leptin communication to fail in the first place (fructose, MSG, etc.). The good news is that you can tackle both issues with one approach—get rid of man-made junk foods! A simple rule of thumb is to avoid any food advertised on TV or in a magazine. Most often these are packaged foods from big food companies, loaded with the very chemicals that disrupt your brain and the hormones we've been discussing in this chapter. Don't be fooled by their deceptive health claims and marketing gimmicks.

In addition to losing body fat and reducing inflammation, you can restore your leptin function by undergoing periods of lower and then higher caloric consumption. This is one more reason for the strategic 5-Day Food-Cycling Formula in the All-Day Fat-Burning Diet, and specifically, the 1-Day Feast.

## THE BRAIN HEALTH AND FAT CONNECTION

Your brain controls everything in your body. It's that simple. It's your body's command central, regulating everything you consciously and unconsciously do. That's why you don't need to think about breathing, keeping your heart pumping, or ensuring that your blood sugar is balanced. Your brain takes care of all that for you. Even conscious activities like lifting your fork or getting up off the couch begin with an impulse from your brain.

As you've seen, much of your ability to lose weight and keep it off is strongly influenced by the health of your brain and its ability to communicate properly with the rest of your body. Its goal is to keep everything inside you in homeostasis (balance). To do that, it must receive the required feedback from various hormones and chemical messengers. If it doesn't, breakdowns occur. To successfully lose weight and keep it off, you cannot overlook the role your brain plays in hunger, mood, cravings, energy, and motivation.

For instance, dopamine is perhaps the most important neurohormone related to your ability to burn fat. It allows us to experience pleasure. We've seen that, without it, animals lack the motivation to do anything. But, as with every hormone in your body, balance is key. Dopamine helps to control energy, and deficiencies can lead to fatigue and carb and sugar cravings. Thus, those with low dopamine function frequently crave sugar and caffeine because of the brain stimulation these "drugs" provide. Unfortunately, the stimulation is short lived, leading to repeated cravings and overindulgence. Over time, continued reliance on these stimulants causes dopamine signaling to weaken, which leads to a vicious cycle of uncontrollable cravings.

Serotonin is a brain neurotransmitter linked to feelings of relaxation and well-being. Ninety percent of all the serotonin in the body is actually found in the gut, where its main job is to control gut movement. In the brain, it's one of the body's appetite suppressants and helps to curb cravings. It makes you feel satisfied even if your stomach is not full. As a result, you eat less and lose weight.

People with very low serotonin levels often have difficulty tasting and may pile more salt on their food. And since our bodies make serotonin only after we eat sweet or starchy carbohydrates, those with low levels often feel unsatisfied if starch is not part of the meal and struggle to follow a low-carbohydrate diet. Continued low serotonin can lead to depression, weight gain, and insatiable cravings for carbs.

Have you ever devoured the bread they give you while you're waiting for the main course in a restaurant? I know I have. By the time the main course comes around, your appetite has been downsized. This blunting of appetite happens not solely because you've eaten 100 calories' worth of bread. It is primarily due to the fact that increased serotonin release put a brake on your appetite—just one more reason why the right carbs are necessary for fat loss. Successful weight loss depends on serotonin to help control food intake.

In Chapter 5, I'll show you some powerful ways to reinvigorate your serotonin levels without taking medications or devouring the wrong carbs, which you'll only regret minutes later. But keep in mind that carbohydrates are an integral part of the All-Day Fat-Burning Diet. The key is to eat the right ones at the right times. I'll show you how to do all that in Part II of this book.

As you can see by now, most of what drives us to take action comes from the brain, from command central and all of the hormones that communicate with it every second of every day. And these delicate hormone levels are easily offset by stress, the wrong exercise, emotional trauma, caffeine, sugar, and poor food choices. This leads to cravings and behavior that oftentimes leads us to question whether we have someone else living inside us. We just don't feel right when our brain chemistry is off. We feel like we've lost control.

The real long-lasting solution to reclaiming control of your body and your health is improving the quality of your diet, eating the right foods at the right times, exercising more intelligently, and allowing your body to properly rest and recover. The result will be a natural correction that rectifies the hormonal imbalances inside your body that are ultimately the real reason you're holding on to fat. Once your metabolism has been reset, your body will operate as it was meant to and you'll transition into burning fat nonstop. This is my hope for you.

Now that you understand all the obstacles that have been getting in your way, it's time to put the All-Day Fat-Burning Diet to work in your life.

# Part II

# 6 Steps to Reset Your Metabolism

## CHAPTER 3

# STEP 1: SET YOURSELF UP FOR SUCCESS

L et's be brutally honest with each other: You don't really want to do any of this, right?

I don't imagine that you particularly want to exercise, and it wouldn't surprise me to hear that you'd rather not follow a meal plan. In fact, I'm guessing if you had to choose between reading this book and curling up to watch a movie with a big tub of hot, buttered popcorn, you'd choose the latter. Don't worry, I'm not offended. I understand. We humans don't like change, especially any that might be considered "self-improvement." It's daunting and disruptive, a Herculean effort of willpower that you'd rather not deal with. There's a reason you've settled into the limiting habits you have now—they were your way of coping with all the stressors that triggered your weight gain in the first place.

If you need proof that positive change is often a lost cause, look no further than your New Year's resolutions. Most of us believe that when the clock strikes 12:00 on December 31, a magical motivational switch will flip in our brains, allowing us to finally lose weight, get organized, or save more money. *This year,* we say, *everything is going to be different.* The stats tell a very different story, and a depressing one at that—45 percent of people set a New Year's resolution, but only 8 percent of them actually achieve success. Despite our lip service to change, most of us don't go much further than halfheartedly mentioning our resolutions to a friend or writing them down, if we do that much. By the time March rolls around, we're right back where we started, if not worse.

None of this is surprising. It's a hard truth about who we are as humans, and it's the very reason the diet industry exists. I want you to know that improving your life doesn't have to feel like such an impossible mission. More than that, I want you to succeed. I'd like to believe this will be the last "diet" book you'll ever read, but I'm not arrogant enough to be entirely convinced. I am 100 percent certain that I can share some important concepts that will make achieving the change you want a much easier task. It comes down to this: Successful change is all about your mind-set.

In 2002, John Norcross, PhD, professor of psychology at the University of Scranton in Pennsylvania, found that readiness to change, or how prepared a person is to enter the action stage of behavior change, is the single best predictor of success in keeping New Year's resolutions. I'm going to double down on that and say it's your best predictor of success at any time, in any aspect of your life. In my experience, it's really all that matters. That's why I no longer bother trying to convince, debate with, or motivate others to change (including my own family members). I only want to help those who are motivated to become better versions of themselves. Since you're reading this book, I believe that includes you!

In his research on New Year's resolutions, Dr. Norcross also found that "resolvers" reported higher rates of success than "nonresolvers." At 6 months, 46 percent of the resolvers were continuously successful, compared to 4 percent of the nonresolvers. This goes to show that the simple act of setting an intention or goal is a big step toward achieving it. As the old adage holds, "All change begins within"; now we have proof. In this chapter, we're going to hardwire your brain to supercharge your success.

# STEP 1: GET CRYSTAL CLEAR

Before a ship leaves its port, the captain must know where it's going. Planes don't leave the gate until the pilots have a crystal-clear flight plan. Do you have a flight plan for your life? Do you know your destination(s)?

If you want amazing results, you have to envision your ideal future. What do you want to achieve? Do you want to lose 10 pounds or 100 pounds? Do you want to reduce your body fat by 5 percent or maybe look like you did 10 years ago? Whatever you want, you need crystal clarity in order to make significant change happen in your life. If your goal is murky, like a pool of dirty water, you'll have a very tough time achieving it.

Let me share two examples from my own life to illustrate the importance of clarity: When I was about 10 years old, I realized I was a really good soccer player. I also loved performing in front of others. That's when I decided that playing pro soccer was definitely something I wanted to do with my life. For as long as I can remember, I would imagine seeing myself playing in front of tens of thousands of people in the best stadiums around the world. For years, I was very clear about what I wanted. That clear vision gave me the drive to train as hard as I did and continually improve myself. Ten years later, I was playing professionally. There were many ups and downs along the way, but I always believed that I could do it. My belief and determination made my vision become a reality.

When I was 26, I was in sore need of a car. I was building a roster of clients all over town, but I was taking the bus and subway to see them. My first step out of this rut was to create a vision board on which I posted the exact car that I really wanted, along with other experiences I wanted in my life. I then took a picture of my collage and used it as the wallpaper on my laptop.

A few months later, I was visiting my mom and she noticed the big image of the car taking up most of my computer screen. When she asked what it was, I told her that I'd created this vision collage to constantly remind me what I wanted in my life. She understood clearly what I was trying to accomplish, and being the great mom that she is, asked if I had taken the car for a test spin. For some reason, I hadn't even thought of that. Thirty minutes later, we pulled up to the dealership. As I stepped onto the lot, a most welcome surprise greeted me: The exact car that had been plastered on my computer's screen was sitting right in front of me! And I mean the exact same car—same year, make, color, rims, everything! It was crazy! Naturally, I took it for a test drive and was blown away. It was so powerful—a little too powerful, actually—so I ended up getting one model down, which was more suitable for my needs.

None of that would have happened had I not been crystal clear about what I wanted. The same goes for you. You need to be 100 percent crystal clear about what you want. What does it look and feel like? What will your daily life be like when it's yours? Get deeply connected to your end result. This same clear intention-setting process has also allowed me to live in the exact house that both my wife and I envisioned for our family for years. Two years before writing my previous book, I created a vision of becoming a #1 *New York Times* bestselling author. I even took an actual *New York Times* bestseller list and put my name and book title at #1. When my previous book, *The All-Day Energy Diet,* was released, it hit #2 on the *New York Times* bestseller list. Pretty darn close, if you ask me.

I don't share this stuff to brag but to illustrate that stuff doesn't just fall into your lap. You need to work damn hard for it. More importantly, you need to know exactly what you're working toward. You need to have a destination. And if that goal is emotionally compelling to you (which it absolutely must be), you will be motivated to take massive action to attain it.

You've likely heard of the law of attraction, though there's a good chance some of you will roll your eyes when you hear those words. The idea holds that if you focus intently on your deepest desire, the universe will conspire to make it come true. I can see how it sounds a bit "New Age-y," but I know from experience that it works. However, I also know that you must consistently focus and act on your initial vision. That's what really makes the magic happen.

To get started, get very clear about exactly what you want. Once you can see it and feel it, write it down and attach a deadline to it—otherwise it's simply a pipe dream that might happen "someday," a day that may never come. Review your goal every single day. Keep it visible. Attach images to it if you like and post it on your bathroom mirror or your fridge. Keep it in your wallet or put it on your smartphone. Repetition is the mother of mastery, so you need to repeatedly show your brain what you want so it can help you make it happen. Moreover, keeping your goal around you at all times will constantly remind you what to work on to make the big picture become real; it's easy to lose focus when life is bewilderingly hectic.

## Nakeisha's Story

"Before I started the All-Day Fat-Burning Diet, I was desperate. I was cranky, mean, angry, and always tired—so tired. I want to have more children, and I knew my weight was one of the barriers I was facing. I blamed my husband for not trying to lose weight, but I had to be honest and admit that I wasn't either. Something had to change.

"I wanted to eat better, but I just resorted to my comfort foods after every disappointment or failed attempt to do better. Food—especially sweets (chocolate is my *favorite*)—took me to my happy place. I knew I needed to change, but I honestly didn't know how. Then, I found Yuri and this program.

"I knew this was a gift, and I wasn't going to waste it. I'm happy to say that I've shed 30 pounds in 63 days—and this is only the beginning. I have plans to walk a 5K with my husband and son, something I would not have done before. I am also looking forward to surprising my parents when I see them in May at my brother's graduation. With the history of diabetes, heart disease, and cancer that we have in my family, I will stand tall and proclaim that I will *not* have diabetes, heart disease, *or* cancer! I *will* be healthy and help my family learn to walk on a healthier path. Thank you, Mr. Elkaim, for giving me tools to be successful for the rest of my life!"

# STEP 2: PLAN AND PREPARE

You're doing nothing less than building a thrilling new version of yourself, and like any master architect, you need a plan. How can you construct You 2.0 without firm guidelines and steps in place?

I believe that the main reason people fail to achieve their goals is because they don't have a solid plan. They may have something fantastic in mind, but they don't prepare for it. For example, how easy is it to have no idea what you're eating for dinner after a long, tiring day? It's all too common. By the time you shuffle through your front door at day's end, you have little to no willpower left to prepare a healthy meal. The next thing you know, you're dialing up for delivery or peeling the plastic off of a microwave meal. Worse yet, you're elbow deep in a bag of potato chips. Sadly, these decisions don't move you closer to a lean, healthy body.

This is why meal planning is so important. By mapping out a week's worth of meals, it becomes ridiculously easy to quickly whip up a tasty, healthy meal whenever you need to, giving your brain and body even more time to relax. Eating isn't something you should have to worry about. In this book, I've given you a 5-Day Food-Cycling Plan that you should follow to the letter—at least for 21 days—to maximize your fat loss. Thousands of other people have, and they've realized incredible results. In fact, many have found themselves continuing to eat according to its guidelines long after their 21 days are up because it's such a completely natural and healthy way of eating and living. You can do the same.

Likewise, if you go to work out without any sense of what you're about to do, I guarantee that your workout will be far less effective than if you know exactly which exercises to do, how many sets and reps, and so forth. Our brains are like laser-guided missiles, and they rely on us for clear direction. Why don't you tell yours what to aim for? Figure out what you're going to have for dinner this week and then get everything you need from the grocery store. If you work out first thing in the morning, get your workout attire ready to go and load your favorite Yuri-guided workouts on your iPod the night before. By making a plan, you can avoid those last-minute pitfalls and excuses. As the old saying goes, "If you fail to plan, then you plan to fail."

## STEP 3: START YOUR ENGINE

How do you feel before you exercise or prepare a meal? Do you go about it with reluctance or a sense of dreariness, or do you feel pumped up and excited about the task ahead? Actually, it's worth asking: How do you feel right now? You might find this line of questioning puzzling, but it's really important. Although it's easy to overlook, your *state* (your physiology, how you feel, etc.) will predict the action you take and thus the results you achieve. Conversely, it can also predict which action you won't take and the results you'll fail to achieve.

I learned this firsthand in the oddest of places—after walking on burning hot coals at a Tony Robbins event several years ago. It sounds crazy, but firewalking is a centuries-old practice that forces you to harness the "power state." If the walker is strong of mind and in the right state, walking the coals—as terrifying as it may be—becomes an easy task. After spending half the day going from a state of panic to priming my mind and body to believe that I could walk on fire, I did it without flinching and without getting burned.

If we can walk on fire, what else can we achieve when we're in the right state? Don't worry, I'm not going to ask you to walk on fire. However, you can think of your continued struggle with weight as the proverbial fire if you'd like. Are you ready to walk all over it? Getting in peak state is simply a matter of getting your body a little more juiced up. It's about revving up your engine. The easiest way to do this is to stand instead of sit—or try smiling instead of frowning, raising your rib cage instead of slouching, taking a deep breath into your belly instead of breathing shallowly.

All of these simple physical shifts improve your emotional state, which puts you into high gear for taking action. Remember, it's very tough to take massive action if you feel depressed. You can't take on the world if you don't feel capable of it. No matter how doubtful you may feel right now, I'm sure you've had moments of sheer joy and confidence when you felt unstoppable. That's what I'm talking about here. As Tony Robbins says, "Emotion comes from motion." To improve your state, simply change the way you use your body. Within seconds, you will feel better and more ready to take on the world—or at least eat better and work out. That's just another reason for being more active throughout your day.

Here's another way of looking at it.

**State → Feelings → Actions → Results**

In her famous TED Talk, social psychologist Amy Cuddy showed that body language doesn't just affect how others see us, but how we see ourselves. She demonstrated how "power posing"—standing in a posture of confidence, even when we don't feel confident—can increase testosterone, lower cortisol levels, and even improve our chances for success in various social settings. You can adopt any of these power poses to improve your state and feel more confident, charismatic, and unstoppable in a matter of seconds.

For instance, instead of standing in a slouched position with your arms crossed, which is a very weak and defensive posture, stand tall with your head high and your arms outstretched like you just won the 100-meter sprint in the Olympics. Go one step further, and get ready to save the world by standing tall with your hands on your hips like Superman or Wonder Woman. As you do this, put a big smile on your face, and you'll supercharge your state even further.

Exercise is a great way to improve your state because it gets your blood flowing and endorphins rushing. You can also get a similar high by simply bouncing around for a few seconds like a boxer before a fight. You can even celebrate your victory in advance by making a celebratory fist pump—nothing can stop you unless you let it! If this all feels a little funny, consider the fact that animals use this same practice to assert themselves and establish dominance. Apes will stand tall and pound on their chests. Bears will rise right up onto their hind legs. Even the smallest wiener dogs will jump at your legs to make themselves more imposing.

So don't hide. Make yourself big and powerful because, when you do, you put yourself into a state of being ready for action. If you don't feel like working out, raise your hands in the air in celebration or jump around while you listen to the theme song from *Rocky*. It's impossible not to feel better after that. It's time to get to work!

## STEP 4: GET SOCIAL SUPPORT

Now that you're primed for action, it's time to start thinking about your team. The road to a personal breakthrough can be a lonely one, so I always advise my clients to seek out others who are on a similar quest or have already realized the results they're after. You need to surround yourself with positive people who will support you on your path.

It makes sense, doesn't it? You know how much of a hurdle a few discouraging words can be. When someone makes you feel terrible about yourself, it can seriously hinder or even halt your progress. Thankfully, the reverse is true as well: When you hit a tough spot on your mission, a few encouraging words from someone who can empathize can give you just the push you need to make it through. Everyone needs a sidekick from time to time.

This was confirmed by a study in the *Journal of Consulting and Clinical Psychology*, which found that participants recruited for a weight-loss program with friends had greater weight loss at the end of both 4 months of treatment and a 10-month follow-up than did those without similar support. Of those recruited with friends and given social support, 95 percent completed treatment and 66 percent maintained their weight loss in full.[1] Online groups can also play a supportive role. A 2010 study showed that Internet weight-loss communities (think Facebook groups or forums) played a prominent role in participants' weight-loss efforts. The study found that participants really valued the encouragement and motivation, extra information, and shared experiences inside the group.[2]

Findings like these are a big part of why we've created a private "readers-only" Facebook group. If you haven't yet joined us, please do.

Becoming part of a supportive community that knows *exactly* what you're going through will help you live this program to the fullest. You'll also connect with thousands of other men and women who have already transformed their bodies using the All-Day Fat-Burning Diet. Please don't underestimate what a tremendous help this can be. You'll love it.

For access to our private Facebook group, go to alldayfatburningdiet.com/resources.

If social media isn't your style, then at the very least recruit some friends to join you on this journey. But be careful to choose only those who will elevate you. You become who you spend the most time with, so choose wisely.

## STEP 5: CREATE A WINNING ENVIRONMENT

Environment will always trump willpower. No matter how committed you are to your goals, if you're hiding stashes of chocolate, ice cream, or other tempting foods around the house—no matter how far out of sight—you will eventually eat them. Trust me on this one.

Your personal environment needs to be a *dojo*, streamlined in perfect congruence with who you want to become, not necessarily who you were until now. What got you here won't get you to the next level. My business coach and mentor, Dan Sullivan of Strategic Coach, always says this: "The skills that got you out of Egypt aren't the same skills that will get you to the promised land." What you then have to ask yourself is this: How can you continue to refine your get-fit skills if you've booby-trapped your home with apple pies and cheese puffs?

We constantly hear that it's important to practice discipline, but we can only rely on our self-control for so long. Willpower is like a battery that dwindles away with continued use; at a certain point, it's completely drained, and that's when the bingeing commences. For this reason, it's important not to sabotage yourself by having unhealthy foods around. Furthermore, relying on willpower has unwanted physiological effects as well.

It's not common knowledge, but self-control uses up your blood sugar, a limited energy source. A study done by the American Psychological

Association showed that low levels of blood glucose after an initial self-control task predicted poor performance on a subsequent self-control task.[3] So if you dodged that ice cream sundae for dessert at lunchtime, it will be that much harder to say no to chocolate cake after dinner! Makes sense, doesn't it? This is why we crave sugar and sweets when we're stressed or have had a long day resisting temptations and performing other acts of self-control. We're wired that way.

Although you can train your willpower, it's much like a muscle that can be temporarily fatigued. Thus, if it's fatigued when you need it most and your environment is not set up for your success, failure is imminent. I'm sure you know what I mean. How many times have you woken up in the morning with the best of intentions to eat healthy and get in a workout only to find yourself by day's end glued to the couch, devouring a plate of cookies? It happens to the best of us, and now we know why.

The key is to set up your environment so that it supports you in your moments of weakness. Sure, it's easy to eat clean when you're full of energy and motivation in the morning, but you really need your environment to come through for you when you're feeling grumpy and tired, perhaps later in the day. Your environment can be anything from your kitchen or your entire home to your car and even your office. The sneakiest one is the office-away-from-the-office: the coffee shop. That's where most moments of weakness occur: hunched over a laptop, typing away and snacking on a sugary muffin between keystrokes. Bars and nightclubs are just as dangerous. If you make it a point to hang out anywhere there's a bartender, you're much more likely to have a stiff drink.

One of the best things you can do to combat this is to de-clutter your surroundings. A cluttered environment leads to cluttered thinking and less than ideal behavior. I don't personally know many successful people who live like hoarders. Everything is neat and clean in their world. I do my best not to judge, but I can almost predict your quality of life by the state of your surroundings. If your car is littered with junk and your house is a complete mess, then that's a reflection of you as an individual.

To let go of the weight, you need to let go of the junk. So, go through your fridge and pantry and toss all the packaged junk that won't support your health and weight-loss goals. Dump the sauces loaded with hidden sugars and MSG. Trash those chips and crackers laced with inflammatory vegetable oils. The chocolates hiding at the back of your cupboard? Give them to a neighbor or throw them in the garbage. Instead, fill your refrigerator and cupboard with fresh produce, nuts and seeds, fit fats, and clean proteins.

Next, attack any mess in your house. Imagine you're a drill sergeant instructing the troops. If there's anything on your counters that doesn't need to be there, put it where it belongs. Organize your drawers and fridge shelves. If you're thorough, you're bound to end up with a pile of things you don't need and should donate to charity. Having less is certainly more. What you'll find is that as you clean up your environment, you will feel better about yourself and more motivated to improve other areas of your life, too.

Remember, how you do anything is how you do everything. If your environment is a mess, your life is likely a mess as well. A clean house leads to a clean body. In this process, you also have to be efficient and realistic. You want to make sure you're eating healthy foods, but the more work and time required to make a food, the less likely you will be to eat it. This is where planning comes into the picture again; when you have some time, cut up your favorite veggies and make some fresh hummus. Have them ready to go in your fridge so that when you get home after a long day, you can put them out on the counter and snack on them.

## STEP 6: TAKE MASSIVE ACTION

The final step to burning fat, improving your health, and achieving anything else you want in life is to take massive action. Nothing replaces action. *Nothing.* You can believe in the law of attraction all you want, but if you just sit around doing nothing, guess what? Nothing will happen. Action creates attraction. Yes, visualization and focusing on your goals are important, but only if they prompt you into action.

Action is also the very best way to conquer your fears. Don't laugh, but I used to be deathly afraid of big spiders. Just seeing a picture of one would make me shudder. My way around this was to do something that would have sent me into apoplectic shock when I was younger: I held a spider, right in my hand. If you're scared of working out, the best thing you can do is to work out (properly). You'll quickly realize that it isn't all that bad and the rewards it yields are incredible.

As we've learned, change can be difficult. We all want that magic bullet, but unfortunately, change doesn't work that way. It's helpful to understand the specific journey that unfolds between taking an initial action and finally realizing your dreams. Dan Sullivan powerfully hit it home for me more than a year ago when he outlined his "4 Cs," a framework for the change process, from idea to realization.

The first C represents *commitment*, or as I like to think of it, the stage where you finally say, "Enough is enough!" You simply can't live as you have up until this point, and something has to change. In your case, you picked up this book, which is a commitment to burning more fat in a healthy and sustainable fashion. Well done for committing— that's huge! The second C represents *courage*. This is a crucial step toward bridging the gap between wanting something and developing the skills or capabilities to attain it. As Dan famously says, "Fear is peeing your pants. Courage is what you do with wet pants."

Building courage into the process is helpful because it reminds you that there will be times when you feel scared or doubtful. Courage is needed to get you through those tough times. Most people fail on a diet or any new endeavor because they think it's going to be easy and that immediate change will occur. When immediate results do not occur—which is the reality for most people—they just droop like a wilting flower and call it a day. Courage is needed to power through that initial disappointment. It's what ultimately leads you to results beyond your wildest dreams.

On the flip side of courage is *capability*, the third C. By taking consistent action—be it eating well, exercising more intelligently, or following a solid sleep schedule—you are creating new habits that are the key to pushing you past the finish line. The more you take action, the easier it is to keep going. You've built up terrific momentum, which is simply a series of better habits that automatically move you in the direction of your goals. You've now become a highly capable person

## Deborah's Story

Sometimes it's the little things that make all the difference in the world.

After Deborah had her first baby at 37 years old, she was stricken with Hashimoto's thyroiditis, a condition in which your immune system goes to war against your thyroid. In this case, it made Deborah pack on a frustrating and embarrassing 20 pounds.

Rather than wallow in her misfortune, however, Deborah went straight to work. As a holistic health care provider, she already had a healthy diet, but she went further by gradually reducing or cutting out her intake of sugar, gluten, dairy, and soy. On top of all that, she started a regular workout regimen.

She did lose weight, but something still wasn't quite right. She wasn't looking or feeling like herself, despite all of her hard work.

When Deborah came across the All-Day Fat-Burning Diet, she committed to her health even further, tweaking her already-healthy lifestyle to fall firmly in line with these new protocols.

The results say it all: In 63 days, Deborah went from 159 pounds to 144 pounds, also reducing her waist from 36 to 31 inches, a whopping 5 inches!

and likely experienced consistent fat loss, improved fitness, and better eating and lifestyle habits. By this point, even if you are derailed by some life event, you know you have the capability to get back on track. You know you can lose weight again and, hopefully, keep it off this time.

There's no way around it: You've got to put in the work. However, as daunting as that may sound, it's *how* you put in the work that makes all the difference. If you follow the steps I've outlined here, it becomes a much easier process. I strongly believe that our level of happiness is directly related to our ability to get stuff done. When we do work that produces great results, we feel good about ourselves, and that builds further momentum.

The development of capability finally leads to the fourth C: *confidence.* It's an unshakable belief in yourself that can only be gained by proving yourself *to yourself.* Impressing others is fleeting; impressing yourself can change your life. This 4-C framework reminds us that there's a specific process between dream and reality. That gap is largely bridged by having the courage to take consistent action. Of all the things I've shared with you in this book, this is what really counts. Sure, the dietary and exercise protocols are important, but unless you have the inner game figured out and are committed to taking action, then nothing will ever work.

Even if you doubt yourself, I know you've got the chops to create the body of your dreams. You've already demonstrated you have what it takes by exercising your commitment to read this far into the book. Just take the next step and keep going. In fact, put the book down right now and do 10 pushups to create some positive momentum. I'm serious! Don't worry about failure, because the only time you truly fail is when you give up, so as Winston Churchill famously said, "Never, ever, ever give up."

If you don't lose 5 pounds in the first week, don't beat yourself up or criticize this program. It's only been 1 week! In a 100-year life span, that week represents a mere 0.02 percent of your time on this planet. You certainly didn't pack on the weight you want to lose in that short a time.

Admittedly, you can achieve very fast transformations with this program, especially if you have a lot of weight to lose, but never forget that this is a lifelong journey for you. And the journey isn't really about the number of pounds you want to drop, but the healthy, fulfilling life you want to live. You don't want to lose all this weight only to gain it back a few indulgent months later. Just as you've committed to this book, commit to your new, superstar life. Even if you don't realize it, you already have! I think that's certainly worthy of a fist pump.

## CHAPTER 4

# STEP 2: REBOOT YOUR KITCHEN

If you have cable television, you've no doubt watched those home-remodeling shows in which construction and design experts completely overhaul outdated homes, much to the delight of their cheery, grateful owners. That's what we're about to do with every aspect of your life, from the stuff in your fridge to your morning routine, and even your body itself.

The aim here is to put you through a hard reset, much as you would a computer that's acting buggy. From my days at university until now, I've never stopped learning about the human body, yet the more I learn, the more I realize that underneath all the stress, junk food, and lack of quality exercise inherent in modern life, our bodies still have the same factory settings as when humans first walked the earth. That's what we're aiming to get back to, step by careful step, so you can get back to being lean and healthy—as nature intended.

Take a second to think back to those times. Men, women, and their Paleolithic-era tribes had only a few basic needs in order to survive—food, water, shelter, and the ability to reproduce. They didn't have fancy condos, workplace cubicles, fully stocked kitchens, or a local

Starbucks to drop by every morning on the way to the hunt. Contrast that with today's modern world: You're jolted out of bed by an annoying alarm clock—sometimes before the sun even rises—and eat a breakfast that more often than not comes from a box. Then you hop in your boxy car and drive to work, where you spend most of your day imprisoned in a cubicle, sitting and chugging cups of coffee and sugar-filled treats to make it through your list of never-ending tasks. You finish the day completely exhausted and return home for dinner—which, more often than not, comes from a box. Is it any wonder our bodies have rebelled?

Undoing this dreadful pattern is not easy, but I've calibrated this plan to make it a smooth process for you. It will certainly take some work on your part, but if you weren't up for the challenge, you wouldn't have picked up this book. By the end of these 3 weeks, you will have successfully remodeled your life. Like many of those home makeover shows, we have to start where you spend a great deal of your time at home: the kitchen.

## THE "FAT AND FILTHY" FOODS

Let's get one thing straight: You will not be eating bird food on the All-Day Fat-Burning Diet. This plan is full of tasty meals that don't deprive you of any enjoyment at mealtime, although some foods are a definite no-no. By simply eliminating them from your diet, you'll already be making tremendous progress toward losing the pounds that are weighing you down.

These foods include:

Dairy

Wheat

Rye

Oats (unless gluten-free)

Refined sugar

Agave syrup

Caffeine

Most foods that come in a box or package

Fast foods (McDonald's, KFC, etc.)

Soy

Vegetable oils (canola, sunflower, safflower, corn, soybean)

# FOODS THAT CREATE A HEALTHY FOUNDATION

What you need to power you through this transformation is better fuel in your tank—fresh, high-quality, whole food. The crap food you've been eating derails your long, tiring day, so it's essential that we replace it. That said, it can be quite confusing trying to figure out just what's healthy and what isn't. We are continually misled by the latest dietary and fitness advice—much of which is nonsense. Sadly, there's research to support almost any claim, which doesn't make matters any easier.

The result is that many people continue to eat junk once they embark on their fitness mission, lured by comforting labels such as "low-fat" this and "low-calorie" that, not realizing that the other ingredients in these food items are complete garbage. Don't forget that one of the major reasons so many people are struggling with weight these days is all the processed junk they're eating. As tasty as it may be, it ends up disrupting their fat-burning hormones and impairing normal brain function.

Most foods you find in a box or package are engineered to make you crave them. They've been cleverly designed with just the right amounts of sugar, fat, and salt to trigger the reward center in your brain. Even if they're lower in calories, these foods are often loaded with artificial additives and other dubious ingredients that do much damage to our health in the long run. Evaluating foods strictly on the basis of their calorie content causes us to miss the bigger, more important picture.

Do you think 1,000 calories of broccoli has the same effect in your body as 1,000 calories of French fries that have been deep-fried in rancid oil? Sure, they both have the same *quantity* of calories, but the *quality* of these calories is a universe apart. Broccoli provides a vast spectrum of nutrients like sulforaphane and indole-3-carbinol, both of which improve detoxification, aid in weight loss, and even prevent some cancers. What health benefits do French fries provide? When you find an answer, please let me know because I've yet to find one.

I'm not a food Nazi. I'm not here to tell you that you can never have

French fries, pizza, or ice cream again. I'll indulge in those "treats" myself on occasion, but certainly not on a daily or even weekly basis. If you're really serious about shedding that weight, I'd strongly suggest that you follow the "clean and lean" eating principles I'm about to share with you—at least for the following 21 days. After that, you can decide how to proceed. In case you're wondering, I've seen some people follow the 5-day plan you're about to discover while still eating common junk foods throughout, everything from pizza to brownies. Although they did lose some weight, it wasn't much compared to the weight lost by those who stayed "clean and lean."

## The Fantastic Four: Why "Clean and Lean" Foods Speed Fat Loss

Eating isn't just about avoiding artery-clogging, fat-building foods; it's about eating foods that turn your body into the Concorde. "Clean and lean" foods provide four essential benefits that we rely on in this program. They will drastically lower inflammation in your body, stabilize your blood sugar levels, speed toxins out of your body, and—in the case of most of the vegetables—alkalize your body.

Your body cannot become a healthy, 24/7 fat-burning machine without these four elements in place. That's why the foods that provide these beneficial effects are at the very foundation of the All-Day Fat-Burning Diet. They are essential for reversing the litany of problems I shared with you in the first section of the book.

## THE ALL-DAY FAT-BURNING DIET "CLEAN AND LEAN" FOODS

Every food contains fat, protein, and carbohydrate in addition to hundreds of smaller micronutrients. For that reason, it's not quite accurate to classify one food as just "fat" and another as "protein." For our purposes, however, I've put the foods into each category based on their predominant macronutrient. For instance, certain high-fat nuts are in the Fit Fats section, while other high-protein nuts are listed as Clean Proteins.

## Fit Fats

Most of the best sources of healthy, "clean and lean" fats come from the plant kingdom. (An exception: the highly inflammatory vegetable oils on our earlier "fat and filthy" list.) Here are the fit fats you will eat more of on this plan.

| | |
|---|---|
| Coconut oil | Coconut |
| Olive oil | Walnuts |
| Hemp seed oil | Brazil nuts |
| Flax oil | Macadamia nuts |
| Fish oil | Pistachios |
| Algae oil | Cashews |
| Coconut milk | Pecans |
| Butter | Pumpkin seeds |
| Ghee | Sesame seeds |
| Avocado | Sunflower seeds |
| Olives | |

## The "But" in Butter

You'll recall that I don't recommend drinking milk or eating cheese or yogurt made from cow's milk, as dairy products create inflammation inside the body. If you absolutely must have some yogurt or cheese, then choose a goat's milk version since most people seem to tolerate it better. You can also easily replace cow's milk with almond milk, hemp milk, or even coconut milk, all of which are much healthier for you. The only exception I've made to the dairy rule in this book and in my life is butter.

Butter is essentially milk fat with smaller amounts of protein, which means it does still contain allergy-causing proteins, however, so if you have a milk allergy or sensitivity, you may want to steer clear. In such cases, choose healthy coconut oil or even clarified butter.

Clarified butter (also known as *ghee*), most commonly used in Indian cuisine, is produced by melting butter and allowing the components to separate. The water evaporates, some solids float to the surface and are skimmed off, and the remaining milk solids sink to the bottom and are left behind when the butter fat (then on top) is poured off. Because of this, ghee has negligible amounts of lactose and casein, making it a better butter option for most people. As with anything, the source is most important. Whether choosing regular or clarified butter, please do your best to find a grass-fed and organic source. After all, the butter is a reflection of what the cow ate. You certainly don't want to be ingesting years' worth of pesticide residues and hormone injections.

And if you're scared about the fat in butter, don't be. First, you won't be eating buckets of the stuff on a weekly basis but instead using it (optionally) in some of the recipes in this book. You'll also use it for general cooking purposes since it's very stable under heat. Second, butter and pretty much all saturated fats got a bad rap due to one

## Lisa's Story

Lisa's results say it all. I have been so inspired by her progress, especially considering what she was up against: type 2 diabetes, a personal financial crisis, and a chronically ill adult child. When she started the program, her stress level was so high she could barely sleep at night; however, she stuck through it all, and here she is: 9 pounds lighter in just 3 weeks.

Her improvements read like a laundry list: "After 21 days on this plan, I can confidently affirm that my energy is better, my sleep is better, and I no longer wake up with a headache every morning," says Lisa. "My strength is better, and my blood sugars are amazingly better."

What's more, she's been in the trenches on her own.

"I have been able to resist temptation; the chips, ice cream, and baguettes that my husband buys for himself and our last child at home have not even been an issue for me, even on the fast days. I feel sad for them, but focused for myself.

"A huge part of this, I believe, is the exercise component of this program. Other programs might say to exercise, but having the days and times and exercises all spelled out for me makes this whole plan work. I feel stronger and healthier, and success builds on success. The proof is in the pudding."

flawed study by the famous American scientist Ancel Keys more than 50 years ago, which triggered the entire low-fat craze that still persists to a great degree today.[1]

Keys's "Seven Countries Study" showed that the risk and rates of heart attack and stroke were directly and independently related to the level of total serum cholesterol, which was, according to Keys, largely caused by saturated fat and cholesterol from the diet. The study was so popular that his findings and suggestions were adopted by the American Heart Association and even the American government. Keys also found himself on the cover of *Time* magazine in 1961, celebrated as the leading light in the world of diet and health.

It's a pity his studies were thoroughly unsound. He pegged saturated fat and cholesterol as the villains in the modern diet but somehow forgot to look at other important cardiovascular enemies, like sugar. Furthermore, Keys based his studies on just six countries out of 21 for which data were available. Analysis of all 21 countries made the link between fat intake and heart disease far from significant. He omitted it anyway.

It's shocking that the medical community and food industry adopted their low-fat recommendations based on such misleading science. Thankfully, we now know better. Take, for instance, a 2014 review of his studies, which found that "current evidence does not clearly support cardiovascular guidelines that encourage high consumption of polyunsaturated fatty acids and low consumption of total saturated fats."[2] So fat isn't the problem. The *wrong kind* of fat is.

Butter isn't the bad guy when it comes to heart disease. Trans fats and rancid vegetable oils (canola, corn, soybean, etc.) are the true culprits because of the inflammation they create inside the body, which leads to elevated levels of dangerous LDL cholesterol.[3] Funny enough, butter is actually good for you.

Butter, especially from grass-fed cows, is a significant source of conjugated linoleic acid (CLA), a special type of fat shown to have powerful anticancer, antidiabetic, and weight-loss-promoting benefits.[4] Butter is also the highest source of butyric acid, or butyrate (from the Greek word for butter, *boutyron*), a very short-chain fatty acid that gets fermented in the small intestine and feeds your healthy gut bacteria, reducing inflammation and doing wonders for the health of your gut.

When fed a high-fat diet of lard and soybean oil, some strains of mice overeat, gain fat, and become insulin resistant. However, a 2009 study in the journal *Diabetes* showed that the simple addition of butyrate to their diet eliminated the harmful metabolic effects of the high-fat diet on such mice. The butyrate-fed mice remained lean, avoided metabolic problems, and showed increased energy expenditure via increased body heat production. The butyrate also substantially increased the function of their mitochondria, the tiny powerhouses of each cell in the body.

Butyrate lowered blood cholesterol levels in these mice by approximately 25 percent and their triglycerides by nearly 50 percent. It lowered their fasting insulin by nearly 50 percent and increased their insulin sensitivity by nearly 300 percent. And it even caused their food intake to decline by roughly 20 percent after 10 weeks. The mice simply didn't want to eat as much food.[5]

This is obviously my own anecdotal theory, but maybe butter plays a role in why French people don't seem to gain as much weight as Americans. I lived in France when I played pro soccer in my early twenties. I can tell you that butter is like oxygen to them. They aren't fussing about it. On this side of the Atlantic, we've been scared off butter and told that man-made, trans fat–laden margarine is healthier for us. It is not. Butter really will not make you fat, especially when consumed in the small quantities that you'll enjoy in this plan's recipes. And it has many health benefits.

## Clean Proteins

We're on a mission to restore you to your most natural state; for this reason, the meat in your diet should meet the same standards. You don't want to be overburdened, stressed out, and pumped full of medication, so the animal that ends up on your plate shouldn't have been either. Whenever possible, choose animal proteins from organic, wild, free-range, or grass-fed sources. Most commercially raised animals are pumped full of hormones and antibiotics and fed unnatural foods like soy and grains, which degrade their health and end up adding to your body's toxic load.

Although this list does contain a lot of animal protein options, I would strongly encourage you to seek out more vegetarian protein sources. Plant-based proteins are less acidic and usually contain a greater array of nutrients than their animal counterparts. The only dilemma with plant proteins is that they also come with more carbohydrates. For the most part, that's not a problem, but when the program calls for you to eat fewer carbs than usual, you'll want to cut back a bit. We'll address this further in the next chapter. Meanwhile, here are your clean proteins.

| | |
|---|---|
| Hemp seeds | Game (bison, etc.) |
| Almonds (raw or soaked) | Pork |
| Lentils (cooked or sprouted)* | Ham (nitrate-free) |
| Black beans* | Bacon (nitrate-free) |
| Navy beans* | Eggs |
| Pinto beans* | Salmon (wild caught) |
| Chickpeas (garbanzo beans)* | Sardines |
| Cannellini beans* | Anchovies |
| Kidney beans* | Trout, rainbow |
| Chicken (free range) | Shrimp |
| Beef (ideally, grass fed) | Lobster |
| Turkey | Crab |
| Lamb | Oysters |

*Indicates a higher presence of starchy carbs in addition to its protein content.

## Starchy Carbs and Fruits

These are the healthy starchy carbs and fruits that I recommend. Obviously, you would limit them on your Low-Carb Days.

| | |
|---|---|
| Sweet potatoes | Beets |
| Yams | Carrots |
| Potatoes | Parsnips |

| | |
|---|---|
| Turnips | Figs |
| Quinoa | Oranges |
| Buckwheat | Grapefruit |
| Amaranth | Grapes |
| Millet | Melon (all types) |
| Gluten-free oats | Pineapple |
| Tomatoes | Mango |
| Bananas | Papaya |
| Apples | Lemon* |
| Pears | Lime* |
| Berries (all types) | |

*Considered a garnish more than a consumed fruit, these are exempt from serving size simplifier guidelines.

## Fibrous Veggies

This class of veggies is the secret to amazing health. You can enjoy these nutrient-rich vegetables to your heart's content on any day within our 5-Day Food-Cycling Formula except for your 1-Day Fast.

| | |
|---|---|
| Spinach | Cabbage |
| Kale | Bell peppers |
| Swiss chard | Celery |
| Lettuce and salad greens | Mushrooms |
| Collard greens | Sprouts (bean, broccoli, etc.) |
| Arugula | Cucumber |
| Broccoli | Zucchini |
| Cauliflower | Eggplant |
| Brussels sprouts | |

## Optional Foods

These foods can be eaten in small amounts on this program. They won't hurt you, nor will they derail your fat-loss efforts. Yet I would keep them to a minimum since high amounts will not support your health and weight-loss goals.

Goat's milk and yogurt          Honey

Maple syrup

## An Important Consumer Awareness Message Regarding Beans, Legumes, and Gluten-Free Grains

I love a good black bean chili on a cold winter day. I also love adding sprouted lentils to my salads or sipping on a thick and filling lentil soup. And why not, considering that beans and legumes provide so many health benefits, including high amounts of protein, fiber, and low-glycemic carbohydrates?

The trouble is that, for years, many people (especially within the Paleo community) have demonized beans, legumes, and even gluten-free grains because they contain "anti-nutrients" like phytic acid. The thinking is that phytic acid binds itself to minerals such as iron, calcium, and magnesium and leeches them out of your body. In *The Adrenal Reset Diet*, Dr. Alan Christianson puts this argument to rest.

> Phytic acid does bind with minerals, but it does so within the foods before you eat them. Therefore, it cannot take minerals out of your body that you have already absorbed. The main negative factor involving phytic acid is that it hampers the absorption of iron in the foods that contain phytic acid. This means that if your only source of iron is plants, as in eating beans and spinach, you may not absorb enough iron. But if your diet includes animal sources of iron, such as dark-meat poultry and red meat, you will absorb the iron just fine, even if you eat foods with phytic acid, such as beans, in the same meal.[6]

If you're scared to eat beans and legumes, then hopefully this information will put your mind at ease.

Aside from the fiber, protein, and good carbs they contain, beans and legumes have some really neat, lesser-known benefits. For instance, white beans like navy beans and cannellini are the most abundant plant-based source of phosphatidylserine. This tongue-twisting component of your cell membranes plays a key role in communication between your cells, and specifically in the programmed death of damaged cells.[7] It basically sweeps the bad cells out.

The anti-bean brigade might be surprised to learn that a 2014 meta-analysis in the *American Journal of Clinical Nutrition* found that legume consumption was inversely related with heart disease among the 501,791 individuals studied. Basically, eating more legumes lowered people's risk of heart attack.[8] Hmmm. I wonder why? Could it be because they're so full of fiber and high-quality carbohydrates? Another 2014 review of the literature set out to examine the effect of non-soy legume intake on markers of inflammation in the body, including C-reactive protein. The researchers compiled all the studies on the topic and found that nonsoy legume consumption contributes to reductions in C-reactive protein concentrations. In English, that means less deadly and fat-inducing inflammation in the body![9]

These findings have been supported by previous research, like a 2011 study in the *European Journal of Nutrition* in which overweight and obese subjects were randomly assigned to either a calorie-restricted, legume-free diet (the control group) or a calorie-restricted, legume-based diet (the legume group) for 8 weeks. The legume group was asked to eat only four weekly servings (160 to 235 grams total per week) of lentils, chickpeas, peas, or beans in addition to their regular food. At the end of the 8-week study, the legume group saw significant reductions in inflammatory markers, such as C-reactive protein. They also lost more weight and benefited from significant improvements in blood lipid profiles and blood pressure, compared with the control group.[10]

So can we lay this bean and legume issue to rest? It's quite clear that they facilitate weight loss and are great for your cardiovascular health. It turns out that old playground song is true after all.

*Beans, beans, good for your heart . . .*

You know the rest. If you don't, give it a Google. We're moving on.

## Superstarches

As of this writing, carbs are considered the enemy in the traditional weight-loss doctrine. Starches of any sort are villainous substances that stick to your hips and fill you out all over. They are to be avoided at all costs.

That's actually not true at all, and there are, in fact, superstarches (or "fat-burning fibers," if you like) that will accelerate your fat loss. You heard that right.

These starches fall under the heading of resistant starch. It's a type of fiber not digested in your stomach or small intestine, proving hardy enough to reach your gut (colon) intact. Thus, it "resists" digestion and, unlike other carbs, does not spike your blood sugar or insulin level. Furthermore, it doesn't provide any significant calories. Yes, this is

## Michelle's Story

"During my pregnancy, I developed preeclampsia and gained approximately 60 pounds. Having always been thin, I was very frustrated when I could not lose the weight, even with 5 to 7 hours of exercise a week. My daughter turned 3 and I still was carrying around pregnancy weight, plus I started to develop digestive disorders. I thought there was nothing I could do. Then I read *The All-Day Energy Diet*.

"When I started this diet, I had already had great success with the All-Day Energy Diet. I had gone from 187 pounds to 163 pounds in 4 months. However, I still had many cravings and slowly increased my cheat meals, and I was consuming alcohol and caffeine. I felt I wanted to do something extra to get back on track. Once I decided to give up coffee and alcohol completely, it was not as difficult as I'd thought. In general, I sleep better and have more energy than before. I have become accustomed to healthy food and prefer my morning smoothie to the bagel and cream cheese I used to have most mornings. I love that I feel in control of what I eat, and I am consistently making better choices. I don't feel that my cravings for sugar, caffeine, alcohol, and wheat products control me any longer.

"I am fitting into clothes that I wore before I was pregnant, and I'm down to 151 pounds. I can see more muscle and less fat and am starting to feel like myself again!"

actually a real thing. What makes it even more special is the fact that it's digested only by the good bacteria in your gut. In other words, it is not food for you, but for your gut flora. We call this amazing food a *prebiotic*.

The normal human gut has hundreds of bacterial species, some good and some not so good. The overall number and proportion of each type have profound effects on our health and well-being. Research has shown that resistant starch selectively stimulates the good bacteria in our intestines, helping to maintain a healthy balance of bacteria.[11] When you eat resistant starch, the good bacteria in your gut feed on it and produce short-chain fatty acids (through fermentation), the most significant of which is butyrate, which you might remember from our discussion on butter. It has numerous beneficial effects on intestinal and overall health.

Butyrate is important because it's the ideal energy source for the cells that line your intestinal tract. There, it acts as a powerful anti-inflammatory agent for your delicate intestinal cells and improves their integrity by decreasing intestinal permeability (bye-bye, leaky gut) and therefore keeping toxins in the gut and out of the blood-stream.[12, 13] But wait, there's more.

Butyrate, produced by resistant starch consumption, also decreases inflammation throughout your body because whatever amount your intestinal cells do not use enters your bloodstream. It is then sent to your liver, from which it spreads throughout the body, where it exerts additional anti-inflammatory effects.

The most abundant food sources of resistant starch are:

- Green (unripe) bananas
- Plantains
- Cooked and cooled parboiled rice or legumes
- Cooked and cooled potatoes

You can also supplement with unmodified potato starch (not potato flour), as it is one of the best sources of resistant starch, with approximately 8 grams per tablespoon. Plantain and green banana flour are also excellent sources of resistant starch. Rotating among all three might be your best option to get a full spectrum of various resistant starch strains. These supplemental options don't have much flavor and can thus easily be added to cold or room-temperature water or mixed into your smoothies. To maintain the benefits of resistant starch, these sources should not be heated above 130°F.

If you choose this supplemental route, start with small doses of about ¼ to ½ teaspoon once daily and gradually increase the amount over time. If you don't experience any of the gas or bloating that can occur when consuming resistant starch—or all fiber, for that matter—as your gut flora changes and adapts, you can likely increase your dosage. About 4 tablespoons per day is all you need for maximum benefit. If you experience too much discomfort, decrease the amount you're taking for a few days until your symptoms resolve, then gradually try increasing it again.

The health benefits of resistant starch usually start to kick in when consuming around 15 to 30 grams daily (equivalent to 2 to 4 tablespoons of potato starch). This may be too much for you to tolerate, especially if your gut bacterial balance is out of whack, but over time it can make a noticeable difference to your health and waistline. A 2005 study in the *American Journal of Clinical Nutrition* compared 4 weeks of supplementation with 30 grams of resistant starch per day with a placebo, and found that it decreased blood sugar, decreased insulin, and increased the ability of the muscles to utilize glucose by 65 percent—independent of any diet or exercise changes.[14] Not too shabby.

## YOUR NEW KITCHEN

By taking a day or two to remove all the junk from your diet and replace it with the beneficial foods I've just listed, you will have taken a massive leap toward the more slender, healthy body you've been dreaming of for such a long time. However, the real magic is yet to begin. You have all the pieces you need, so now you just need to see the big picture they compose before you put them all together. That, my friend, is the heart of this very program, the 5-Day Food-Cycling Formula.

CHAPTER **5**

# STEP 3: FOLLOW THE 5-DAY FOOD-CYCLING FORMULA

Y ou probably won't be surprised to hear this, but you have terrible eating habits.

If it's any consolation, so does almost everyone you know. These days, eating seems to be far more about entertainment and indulgence than nourishment, and the evidence can be seen in our waistlines. The solution is not to stock up on low-fat foods from the supermarket or commit to suffering through a fad diet, but to rewire your entire relationship with food and even hunger itself.

To get you on the right track, we're not only going to address what you eat, but also how often you eat. Don't worry, there won't be any weeklong fasts on this program, but we will get you accustomed to eating only when you're truly hungry. We often have a meal only because the clock tells us it's time to, not because our stomach does. We're putting an end to that.

The notion that we need three square meals a day to properly function is a relatively modern one that emerged from the Industrial Revolution of the mid-1800s. The advent of factory life made long, standardized working days a norm in Western society, and with this shift came the fashion of eating at the beginning, middle, and end of each day. It has been made even worse by food companies that push their cereals and other unnecessary breakfast options on you, making you feel like you "need" to eat breakfast. You don't, especially if you're not hungry in the morning.

There's nothing inherently wrong with three meals a day, but as you'll come to see, sticking to this schedule is not always necessary. In fact, we're going to reschedule your eating according to what I call the 5-Day Food-Cycling Formula. This is the schedule that you're going to follow for the next 21 days, and it's specifically designed to help you shed the excess weight you've been carrying around. Why 21 days? That's really the minimum amount of time it takes to form a habit. You'll quickly see that you can do this for much longer, but 21 days is a great starting point. What's more, during this time period, your relationship with food will evolve, as the plan trains you to eat the foods you truly need when you truly need them, all without sacrificing taste or your enjoyment at breakfast, lunch, or dinner. You can still be a foodie on this program.

## THE BREAKDOWN

This diet is not a low-fat diet, a no-carb diet, or a vegan diet. It incorporates aspects of each, but this diet is based on science, not trends or fitness demagoguery; in fact, I'm hesitant to call this a diet at all.

I don't want to use the word *diet* because this program is not based on deprivation. You'll be eating nourishing, delicious meals that leave you satisfied, whereas following most diets ends up feeling like an ordeal. Even though you will have to put in some work, and there will be a few rough days here and there, this program will ultimately renew you from the inside out.

Every day for the next 3 weeks (and hopefully beyond), you'll be waking up to easy-to-follow guidelines cycling you through the following five daily schedules.

**Day 1:** The Low-Carb Day

**Day 2:** The 1-Day Feast

**Day 3:** The 1-Day Fast

**Day 4:** The Regular-Calorie Day

**Day 5:** The Low-Calorie Day

Let's break down what each of these days looks like.

## DAY 1: THE LOW-CARB DAY

Repeat after me: Not all carbs are bad. To some of you, that might sound sacrilegious, in which case you should repeat the phrase at least three more times.

No-carb and low-carb diets are but the latest in a long line of weight-loss trends dating back to the early 20th century. Why, in the 1920s, even cigarettes were marketed as a way to lose weight! In the 1950s, there was the cabbage diet, which held that eating a bowl of cabbage soup once a day was the way to a slender body. There was also the grapefruit diet and even the ridiculous Hollywood cookie diet that pushed special cookies made with a supposedly fat-blasting blend of amino acids.

However, thanks to the Internet and social media, the low-carb craze has taken hold in popular culture in a way no other diet has before. It was popularized by *The Atkins Diet* and *The South Beach Diet* in the 1990s, but since then has come to be thought of as a general rule for anyone looking to shed fat fast. These villainous carbs, we're told, are inessential nutrients that cause inflammation and spike your blood sugar and insulin, thus causing your body to store fat.

It would be nice if the answer was as simple as that, but it's not. If anything, avoiding carbs like the plague could do your body more harm than good. It's all about determining which carbs are good for you and which aren't and how many of them you really need. Here's the lowdown on carbs once and for all.

As a general rule, eating more carbs than you need for physical activity makes your body less efficient at burning fat. With this in mind, we already know it's important to place a reasonable limit on our carb consumption. Beyond that, we also know that all carbs are not created equal. White, refined carbohydrates—glutenous grains such as breads, pastas, and cereals—are what you probably think of when the word *carbs* is mentioned, but vegetables like broccoli and green peas are also carbs. Can you guess which ones you should and shouldn't be eating?

Indulging in bad carbs can have damaging effects on your blood sugar and insulin levels, which can lead to further weight gain, diabetes, heart disease, and more. Good carbs, however, are an important source of energy for your body. The problem with trying to lose weight by not eating carbohydrates is that most of us require some level of carbohydrates to function at our best over the long term. So given that carbs aren't as bad as they're popularly thought to be, you might wonder why I'm suggesting you restrict carbohydrate intake on some of the next 21 days.

Reducing the amount of carbohydrates in your diet periodically does remain one of the best ways to lose weight. It tends to reduce your appetite and prompts automatic fat loss, without the need for calorie counting or portion control. This means that you can eat until you feel full and satisfied, and still lose weight.

But low-carb diets, in the long run, are no better than any other diet. As you become more active, keeping carbs too low for too long can have disastrous consequences. If you're typically sedentary and carry around quite a bit of body fat, your carbohydrate needs are naturally lower because you're using less energy. As such, you might be able to get away with a lower amount of carbs in your diet. On the other end of the scale, I'm pretty slender, hovering between 7 to 9 percent body fat, which means that if I completely removed carbs from my diet, I would whittle away to nothing in no time. I need carbs for energy, but rather than bingeing on them, I cycle them intelligently. So can you.

For our purposes, if you simply remove the unhealthiest carb sources from your diet—wheat (including whole wheat) and added sugars—then you'll be well on your way to improved health and you'll notice the pounds drop off almost automatically. However, to enjoy the full meta-

## THE MYTH OF THE LOW-CARB DIET

You may notice friends and magazines raving about low-carb diets, but if you follow the science, these diets aren't all they're cracked up to be. In a 2006 study published in the *American Journal of Clinical Nutrition*, subjects were randomly assigned to a low-carb diet (60 percent of energy as fat, 5 percent of energy as carbohydrate) or moderate-carb diet (30 percent of energy as fat, 40 percent of energy as carbohydrate). During the 6-week study, participants were sedentary, and their daily diets were strictly controlled.

Results of the study revealed that those who ate a moderate-carb diet reported significantly better mood and lost about the same amount of weight as those on the low-carb, or *ketogenic*, diet.

Actually, the group who ate a moderate amount of carbs showed a small (but not statistically significant) tendency to lose more body fat as compared with those on a low-carb diet (5.5 kilograms versus 3.4 kilograms in 6 weeks).[1] Both diets improved insulin sensitivity, but the interesting part was that the low-carb diet increased LDL (bad) cholesterol and inflammatory markers, and subjects who were on it felt less energetic.

The results speak volumes, but I imagine that many low-carb fanatics will turn a blind eye. You don't have to.

bolic benefits of short-term low-carbohydrate intake, you need to restrict other carb sources for specific periods of time as well. After all, we want to kick the fat-burning process into high gear. If you're already mourning the lack of carbs in this program, don't worry; you'll be able to enjoy them to the fullest and without guilt on other days. Staggering your carbs (and calories) in this way is part of the magic of the All-Day Fat-Burning Diet.

We're beginning with your Low-Carb Day, as this kicks off the process of fat burning in your 5-day cycle. The main goal on this day is to deplete your glycogen stores, which will in turn make your body turn to fat as its main fuel source.

You'll see that in the 21-day plan we actually start with two Low-Carb Days. This is done purposefully to lower your glycogen reserves (stored carbohydrates) so that your body starts tapping into more of your stored fat for fuel.

Food-wise, we accomplish this by keeping your "net" carbohydrate intake—the amount of carbohydrate remaining after we exclude fiber—below 50 grams. The first thing I'm sure you're thinking is, *What does that even look like?*

Here's a chart showing the net carb content of a few popular, healthy foods.

| FOOD | NET CARBS |
|------|-----------|
| Mango, 1 whole | 45 g |
| Potato, 1 medium | 33 g |
| Oat bran muffin, 1 small | 28 g |
| Banana, 1 whole | 23 g |
| Pear, 1 whole | 22 g |
| Sweet potato, 1 medium | 22 g |
| Apple, 1 whole | 21 g |
| Orange, 1 whole | 14 g |
| Whole wheat bread, 1 slice | 12 g |
| 2% milk, 1 cup | 12 g |
| Carrots, 1 cup | 9 g |
| Broccoli, 1 cup | 4 g |
| Avocado, 1 whole | 4 g |
| Kale, 1 cup (raw) | 1 g |

As you can see from the chart, it's pretty easy to blow through your 50 grams of net carbs with a few pieces of fruit, so on your Low-Carb Day, we're going to focus on eating a lot of vegetables. We'll also be leaning on the secret weapon of your Low-Carb Day: protein. We know that getting plenty of protein has many advantages, as it revs up your metabolism, makes you feel full longer, and helps you retain lean muscle mass. It turns out that these advantages are just as beneficial to the fat-burning process as depleting your glycogen stores.

A 2012 study in the journal *Physiology & Behavior* revealed just how powerful protein can be when it comes to losing weight. Over the course of 1 year, the researchers compared four different dietary conditions.

1. **Normal protein, normal carbohydrate**
2. **Normal protein, low carbohydrate**
3. **High protein, low carbohydrate**
4. **High protein, normal carbohydrate**

Interestingly, the two groups eating the high protein lost the most weight. Furthermore, varying the levels of fats and carbs seemed to make no difference to body composition.[2]

## Low-Carb-Day Food Guidelines

- Your goal is to eat fewer than 50 grams of net carbs on this day.
- Avoid starchy carbs (root veggies, grains).
- Eat protein at each meal.
- Eat fit fats for energy.
- Eat lots of leafy and cruciferous veggies.
- Eat when you're hungry, and stop when you're full.

### Eat Unlimited Amounts of These Foods
**All Leafy Greens**

| | |
|---|---|
| Spinach | Lettuce |
| Kale | Collard greens |
| Swiss chard | Arugula |

## Cruciferous Vegetables

Broccoli

Brussels sprouts

Cauliflower

Cabbage

## Other

Bell peppers

Cucumber

Celery

Tomato

Mushrooms

Zucchini

Bean sprouts

Eggplant

## *Limit the Following Foods*

For reference: 5 to 7 handfuls equal about 50 grams of net carbohydrates

**Visual serving size = 1 cupped handful**

Nuts and seeds

Avocado

## *Avoid These Foods*

For reference: 2 to 3 cupped handfuls equal about 50 grams of net carbohydrates

Root vegetables (squash, sweet potato, beets, etc.)

Dairy*

Wheat and glutenous grains*

Carrots

Healthy nonglutenous grains (quinoa, buckwheat, millet, amaranth, brown rice)

Peas

Corn

All fruit and fruit juices (including smoothies)

*These foods are part of the "fat and filthy" list and should generally be avoided at any time.

Again, we just want to avoid these foods on our Low-Carb Days since they will easily put us over our 50-gram net carb target. It's not that these foods aren't healthy, because many of them are; we're just strategically avoiding them today to bring our carb load down.

## Low-Carb-Day Exercise Guidelines

Speed burst training (5 to 10 minutes)

Follow with 30+ minutes of low-intensity cardio, if desired

For detailed explanations of the exercises throughout the book, see Chapter 6, Step 4: Exercise Using the "LIFT Method" to Burn Fat 24/7.

Before we move on, I thought you'd appreciate answers to some of the common questions I get asked about Low-Carb Days.

### What if I get hungry on Low-Carb Days?

Occasionally, you may feel hungry on your Low-Carb Days. This is because you're avoiding starchy carbohydrates, which fill you up fast and contain a lot of calories. Ride through the hunger by adding more clean proteins, fit fats, and fibrous veggies to your meal. There's no harm in eating some protein, fat, or more salad.

### How many carbs should I eat at every meal?

Even though we're aiming for fewer than 50 grams of net carbs, I certainly don't expect or want you to start obsessing about that. The beauty of this plan is its simplicity. Just follow this one simple rule: On Low-Carb Days, don't eat starchy carbs or fruit, but continue to eat clean proteins, fibrous veggies, and fit fats. Try to remember that when your 1-Day Feast rolls around, you'll be able to eat those starchy carbs and fruits that you've given up today. Simple, right?

### Cheat Tip: Replace Grains with Greens

You'll quickly notice how both the Low-Carb Day and 1-Day Feast are virtually identical: Both call for you to eat lots of protein, veggies, and fat. There's just one simple difference: On Low-Carb Day, we replace the starchy carbs and fruit from your 1-Day Feast with tons of fibrous veggies. In other words, wherever you would have had a starchy carbohydrate (say, brown rice, or maybe a mango), simply replace it with fibrous veggies.

## DAY 2: THE 1-DAY FEAST

Here's when you get to make up for all the carbs you were missing on the Low-Carb Day. If any part of you feels guilty even thinking about this, don't. Your 1-Day Feast is a full-on "eat until you're happy" day. (Technically, you should eat only until you're 80 percent full so you don't feel bloated or totally overload your digestive system.) The main thing here is that you shouldn't worry about eating more than usual. It's fine, and in fact, it's encouraged! As counterintuitive as it sounds, eating more serves a very important purpose in pursuit of faster fat loss.

Having a 1-Day Feast once a week, especially with carbohydrates and fruits thrown back into the mix, is tremendously rewarding. It gives you something to work toward and allows you to let loose and enjoy some of your favorite foods. I can't overstate how helpful this is for your overall morale. It goes a long way toward keeping you on track the other days of the week. More important, this gives your body an opportunity to reestablish proper hormone signaling, damaged by the dysfunctional diet that has left you in your current state. The aim is to load up on healthy food and nourish yourself back to your ideal weight.

Today, that means eating a lot more than you normally would—a full 50 percent more. If you normally eat 2,000 calories a day, on your 1-Day Feast you would aim for about 3,000 calories, with at least 250 grams (or 1,000 calories) coming from carbohydrates. I don't advocate counting calories—which I'll discuss more later in the book—so a really easy way of doing this is to increase your serving sizes by 50 percent. The best way is to simply use bigger cups, bowls, and plates. Or, you can refill your plate or bowl with a second serving, if you still have room in your tummy.

I can't stress this enough, however: Feast only 1 day every 5 days. Attempting to incorporate more than one 1-Day Feast into your week will totally wreck everything you're working toward. And I hate to be an even bigger party pooper, but this is not the "cheat day" that you'll find in other diets. This is not a 24-hour excuse to rip into pizza, ice cream, and cheeseburgers. You're not "allowed" to feast on potato chips and cheesecake. Pigging out on extremely harmful foods filled with sugar, refined wheat, and trans fats will derail any progress you make during the week.

Here's why you don't want to go down that tasty yet terrible road.

1. **Real foods will taste like cardboard.** You've trained your taste buds to respond positively to loads of sugar, salt, and trans fats. Keep it up, and your taste buds won't adapt completely and you won't be able to experience the same satisfaction from real foods.

2. **You'll become a junk food junkie.** Junk foods are downright addictive. If you keep eating them, you'll *crave* more of them. It's that simple. These foods are engineered to light up the reward center in your brain, which means you'll go to great lengths to get more of that good feeling. Abstaining from sugar and junk is the only thing that works for addiction, period.

3. **It's not rocket science: Junk food is bad for you and makes you fat.** Other than to soothe emotional needs and cave into cravings, why else do we eat junk foods? Do they serve any real purpose? Knowing how bad these foods are, no logical human being would willingly eat them. Unfortunately, we are irrational creatures and we do things even when we know they're bad for us.

Junk food normally has a high amount of carbs and a high amount of fat. If you get in the habit of eating crap food on your 1-Day Feasts, your body will be more prone to pack on body fat thanks to the combination of high blood sugar, high blood insulin, and high blood fat. Not to mention that you will mess up your fat-burning hormones even further. You'll end up wasting the time you put into getting in shape and even the money you spent on this book.

There are still plenty of ways you can indulge yourself. In fact, I do it every week. In my house, everyone looks forward to Crepe Saturdays. It sounds sinful, but our crepes are actually quite good for you, as they're 100 percent gluten and dairy free and contain no sugar. We load up each crepe with goodies like banana and almond butter, applesauce and cinnamon, or the occasional sweet treat, such as Nutella (yes, I know) with strawberries, banana, and shredded coconut.

Whatever you choose to eat today, just make sure you eat more of it than you usually would, as long as it's within the day's healthy guidelines. After your Low-Carb Day, your glycogen stores will be depleted and you will naturally be hungrier than usual. Therefore, you need to eat more than usual—ideally, a full 50 percent more. To do so, you can:

- Eat bigger meals more often throughout the day.
- Snack throughout the day.
- Add some liquid nutrition (i.e., a smoothie) between your main meals.
- Enjoy a healthy dessert.

If you need to be sold further on the idea that eating more (plus eating carbs) is actually healthy for you, then consider just what kind

## IF YOU'RE STILL WORRIED ABOUT CARBS

I understand that the mere mention of the word *carbohydrates* may still make you feel 10 pounds heavier, but it really shouldn't. After all, eating healthy carbs can help you lose weight. In fact, restricting them for too long can be quite harmful, often leading to unfavorable changes such as the following:

- Decreased thyroid output
- Increased cortisol output
- Decreased testosterone
- Impaired mood and cognitive function
- Muscle breakdown
- Suppressed immune function

In plain English: Your metabolism slows to a halt, your stress hormones run rampant, and your muscle-building hormones plummet.

If you need to be convinced further, consider a study published in the *International Journal of Obesity and Related Metabolic Disorders* in 1997. With a group of formerly obese women as their subjects, researchers set out to investigate the different impacts of a high-sugar diet, a high-starch diet, and a high-fat diet. The women were assigned to one of the three groups and asked to eat as much as they liked, within their assigned dietary restrictions, for 2 weeks.

After 14 days, women who ate the high-starch diet had a 13 percent lower average caloric intake than those who followed the high-sugar and high-fat diets. The "starch" women also experienced a decrease in body weight and fat mass, while no changes were seen on the high-fat or high-sugar diets.[3]

If that's not an argument for healthy carbs, I don't know what is.

of impact it has on your hormones. No matter what you eat or how much you exercise, if your hormones are out of whack, you'll never lose weight. By eating in this fashion, you're restoring hormonal balance, especially of your precious thyroid hormones, which will help restore your body to its ideal weight.

Without going too deep into the science of why eating more carbohydrates (occasionally) is good for you, here's a quick overview.

- It prevents thyroid function from plummeting, which is important for keeping your metabolic rate highly active to help you burn fat.

- It helps prevent hypothalamic amenorrhea in women—a starvation-related response that impairs normal hormone function, which can result in increased body fat, lower bone density, and impaired fertility.

- It maintains testosterone levels and prevents cortisol from increasing due to extended periods (a few days) of low caloric intake, which helps prevent muscle loss and thus metabolic decline.

- It helps to ensure optimal levels of leptin, the hormone that tells your brain you're full, which prevents you from overeating. Conversely, with caloric restriction, leptin levels fall and you end up bingeing because your brain believes you are starving.

As you can see, carbohydrates play multiple important roles in your body, so they're not something you can simply go without. Choosing to go low carb indefinitely is certainly an option, and you will likely lose a lot of weight, but there's a strong chance you'll end up feeling pretty miserable in the process and regain any lost weight if you choose to reintroduce carbs back into your diet.

## *1-Day-Feast Food Guidelines*

- Eat healthy feast foods ad libitum—as you desire, without feeling guilty.

- Don't binge or stuff yourself; eat until you're 80 percent full, not to the point of discomfort.

- Ideally, eat your biggest meal after you work out.

- If you can't eat more at any given meal, then graze throughout the day (in between meals) on nuts, fruit, or other healthy foods.

The hardest part of this 1-Day Feast is for you to be okay with eating at least 50 percent more food than you're used to. Please remember that this day serves a very important role in keeping your thyroid and hunger/satiety hormones happy.

## Examples of 1-Day-Feast Foods

**Gluten-free grains** like quinoa, millet, amaranth, buckwheat, or oats. With these options you can prepare delicious pancakes, oatmeals, hearty salads, and more. See the recipes in Chapter 10 for examples.

**Starchy carbs**—sweet potato, potato, carrots, beets, parsnips, rice, brown rice, gluten-free grains (see above)

**Fruit**—I generally recommend eating more low–glycemic index fruit like berries, apples, and pears. But for your feast day, feel free to have any fruit you like. Yes, you'll be taking in more sugar (both fructose and glucose), but as long as it's in the form of whole fruit (not juiced), you'll be fine. These fruits can also serve as great postworkout refueling options.

**Nuts**—almonds, walnuts, cashews, pecans, pistachios, etc.

**Legumes**—black beans, chickpeas, lentils, etc.

**Healthy fats**—avocado, olive oil, coconut oil, butter, fish oil, flax oil, hemp oil

**Proteins**—lentils, beans (kidney, navy, etc.), grass-fed beef, free-range chicken, wild fish, eggs, bacon (sure, why not?), hemp seeds, chia seeds, protein powder

Any feast foods you enjoy should *ideally* be gluten free, dairy free, caffeine free, nonalcoholic, unprocessed, and whole-food based. Even though this is a feast day, you still want to ensure good health by eliminating inflammatory foods from your diet. In case you've forgotten, I've included a whole host of delicious recipes in the next part of the book. You don't have to reinvent the diet wheel; I've already done it for you.

If you do lose control and splurge on a pizza night with friends, don't be too hard on yourself. Yes, you will most definitely have set back your weight-loss progress, but hopefully, you'll feel the difference in your body and be compelled not to do it again.

## 1-Day-Feast Exercise Guidelines

If possible, do a full-body and/or interval-training workout 1 to 2 hours before you begin your feast day or before you have your biggest meal of the day.

Your muscles are most receptive to the uptake of carbohydrates (for refueling purposes) and nutrients immediately after a workout. In general, your biggest meal should come after you work out in order to replenish depleted glycogen while minimizing any fat spillover. Please bear in mind that, due to lower glycogen levels from the previous Low-Carb Day, you'll likely feel more lackluster than normal. Do your best to get in a great workout in spite of that.

# DAY 3: THE 1-DAY FAST

Pick up a Bible, Quran, or Torah or look into the annals of religious history and you'll come across many mentions of fasting, and with good reason: It's one of the world's oldest and most effective healing and weight-loss modalities. This might run counter to what you've been told, and almost definitely conjures up thoughts of starvation and suffering. After all, it's not commonly practiced today, but that's a shame, as temporarily abstaining from food can not only give your body a rest but also provide some time for contemplation.

Fasting is not necessarily easy and, in fact, can be considered a form of stress, as it has been shown to increase cortisol levels. Much like exercise, however, it's a positive form of stress with many wondrous benefits. If you find yourself suddenly horrified by reading this, don't be: I'm not asking you to embark on a 40-day or even a 40-hour fast. For this program, you can experience the benefits of fasting by giving your body a rest for up to 24 hours after the indulgence of your 1-Day Feast. This readjusts your tastebuds, reduces cravings, and puts you back in control of the food you eat. Furthermore, it can give you tremendous insight into why you eat the way you do.

Before I continue, let me say that if you suffer from reactive hypo-glycemia or diabetes, you may want to consider eating something small every 2 to 3 hours throughout your 1-Day Fast. For you, it won't actually be a fast day, but rather a low-calorie day. However, if you're relatively healthy, even if you're overweight, I would strongly encourage you to follow the plan as it's laid out. This 1-Day Fast will change your life!

According to a 2005 study in the *Journal of Nutritional Biochemistry*, the beneficial effects of intermittent fasting (and caloric restriction, for that matter) result from at least two mechanisms: reduced oxidative damage and increased cellular stress resistance.[4] Basically, that means that it helps your body to deal with stress! And it gets better—just have a look at the multitude of health benefits documented to occur with repeated 12- to 24-hour fasts.

- Decreased body fat and body weight
- Maintenance of skeletal muscle mass
- Decreased blood glucose levels
- Decreased insulin levels and increased insulin sensitivity
- Increased lipolysis (breakdown of fats) and fat oxidation
- Increased uncoupling protein-3 mRNA (important for the production of energy inside the cell)
- Increased norepinephrine and epinephrine levels
- Increased glucagon levels
- Increased growth hormone levels

I don't know about you, but I've never seen a drug that can do so much good for the human (and animal) body. Each of these benefits contributes to weight loss, and they're all completely free. Plus, giving yourself a break from food for a day or two a week will save you money on your grocery bills. Fasting will not only help you lose weight but allow you to really tune in to your body's hunger messages. After doing a few of these fasting days, you'll feel more in control of your body and your relationship with food. Now, from a weight-loss perspective, this 1-Day Fast coincides with an optional low-intensity cardio workout to create a massive caloric deficit while your body is primed to burn fat. This might actually be the most important day of your weight-loss week.

## Understanding Your Hunger Hormones

I must warn you in advance: The first time you do a 1-Day Fast, you'll probably feel pretty miserable. It's to be expected. It's quite like exercise: The first time you work out, you're guaranteed to feel sore for a few days. But just like exercise, your 1-Day Fast will get a lot easier over time.

The reason it's so uncomfortable is because you're literally reprogramming your main hunger hormone—ghrelin. Ghrelin controls your body's hunger response and serves as a short-term regulator of body weight. Your body's levels of ghrelin are primarily regulated by food intake, increasing when you're fasting or hungry and decreasing when you're fed. Thus, whenever you feel hunger pangs gnawing at your stomach, that's ghrelin getting to work. Ghrelin is also the driving force behind enhanced growth hormone (GH) secretion during fasting, which you'll see throughout this book is a very important hormone for fat loss and muscle preservation.[5] Under conditions of nutritional restriction, GH levels are high, leading to the breakdown of fat to provide the calories your body requires to function.

Thus, GH plays a fundamental role in maintaining metabolic homeostasis and body composition. And GH levels are greatly dependent on the presence of ghrelin. Both hormones play a vital role in maintaining healthy blood sugar and energy balance during fasting. This happens because your body perceives hypoglycemia (low blood sugar) as a stressor. Thus, it mounts a "stress response," which includes the release of the adrenal hormones cortisol and adrenaline, along with growth hormone, to raise blood glucose back to normal levels. Ghrelin helps in this process, as it senses low blood glucose and drives growth hormone release.

Because of these hormonal responses, short-term fasting closely mimics high-intensity exercise. That's one of the primary reasons there's a 1-Day Fast built into your 5-day cycle; every hormonal trigger activated by your 1-Day Fast works in your favor to burn more fat and

## Stine's Story

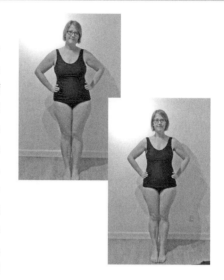

"The start of this diet seems like a life-time ago. For a lot of years I had been stuck in what felt like most areas of my life. I was in a relationship that I knew wasn't right for me but still was hard to end. Over the 14 years of the relationship, I gained a lot of weight. At the worst I was 240 pounds. I managed to get to 192 pounds by myself; however, after ending the relationship a year ago, all those years of stress, the stress of the actual breakup, and a stressful job left me with adrenal burnout. It was so bad I could barely string a sentence together or stand up without severe dizziness, and I ended up being sick for almost 5 months, so any thought of diets was forgotten.

"During this time, I came across the All-Day Fat-Burning Diet, and it just felt right. I am a nutrition student, but due to the stress, I just haven't been able to consistently apply my knowledge. I have been wanting to go wheat and dairy free for a long time, but was not able to take the step.

"What I love about Yuri's programs (not just this book) are that they make sense and are thought through in great detail, especially this

preserve muscle. I personally find that fasting is also a great opportunity to learn a great deal about why you eat the foods you do. Many times the discomfort of fasting is not physiological but psychological. This 1-Day Fast will help you identify some of your conditioned ways of eating and lead to true dietary freedom as you work through them.

## The Easiest Way to Fast

I'm very aware that the mere mention of the term *fasting* terrifies many people, conjuring up images of intense suffering and starvation. They one with the combination of diet and exercise.

"The recipes are fantastic, and I never felt like I was on a diet at all. I have made the recipes for guests several times, and they have always been well received. Even my 4-year-old son is happily eating the food.

"When I started the diet, I was severely addicted to sugar and wheat, but very quickly the cravings subsided. I felt I gained a control I had lacked for years over my diet. It felt like a knot that was loosening, giving me a more relaxed relationship with food. I finally feel like I can hear my body telling me what it needs.

"After 9 weeks on the diet, I can't see myself ever ending it. I love the way both the exercise and diet can easily fit into a busy life. I love the variety of the diet with the mix of low-carb, feast, fast, regular-, and low-calorie days, where you don't get stuck in a rut. This food-cycling plan helped me avoid wanting to rebel against a strict structure (often found in most diets).

"I am now lighter than I've been in more than 10 years. I've gone down two clothes sizes and lost almost 30 pounds! I also feel great and have lots of energy. And I have reopened the lines of communication with my body and feel ready to move on with my life.

"This has been a life changer, not only due to the weight loss, for which I get lots of compliments, but mainly because I have found myself and regained the energy to get out of the rut I was stuck in. Thank you, Yuri, for this opportunity. It has been an amazing journey, which has really just begun."

picture themselves waking up in the morning and starting their 24-hour timer, anxiously counting down the milliseconds until they can have the first bite of their post-fast meal. Others can't even fathom the idea of going a full day without food.

It really doesn't have to be so awful, and there's an approach that actually makes it quite doable. In fact, it's what I do. It's a bit of a cheat, but it doesn't lessen the benefits of your fast, so I say give it a go. The day before your 1-Day Fast is your 1-Day Feast. On that day, about 3 hours after you've enjoyed the last bite of your last meal for the day, start the timer on your 1-Day Fast. For example, if you had a big dinner around 7:00 p.m., your body would be in a "semifasted" state by the time 10:00 p.m. rolls around. Consider that the kickoff of your fast. Hit the sack and sleep for 7 to 8 hours. By the time you wake up, you've completed one-third of your day's fast without batting an eyelash, literally.

If you're anything like me, you might not feel hungry in the morning. There's a good chance this will happen considering how much you stuffed yourself the day before. So much for breakfast. If you can make it to lunch on a few glasses of water, then you've just knocked out 14 hours of your fast. And if you can make it to at least 4:00 p.m., that's 18 hours. You're really on fire at this point. Maybe you can have a cup of peppermint tea as a reward. After all, this is when the massive health benefits from your short-term fast really start to kick in.

At this point, if you really can't take it, you can have a smoothie or smaller meal to break your fast. However, if you really want to win, power through to dinner without taking a bite. Once you reach 10:00 p.m., you've made it. You've successfully completed your fast, and you can go to bed dreaming about breakfast. If you can't wait until morning to eat, I recommend a protein shake with a few carbs about an hour before you go to sleep. That way, you provide essential proteins to your muscles, while keeping your tummy satisfied until morning. The 1-Day Fast isn't easy, but it's not impossible either, and when you stay focused on the benefits, it becomes a lot more doable. Can you do this? I bet you can.

What makes it all a whole lot easier is simply making the decision to do it. Most people have a tough time without food because they're constantly thinking about what they'll eat next. In the middle of a stressful day, fasting just feels like too much to handle, as the satisfaction that comes from a delicious meal—even one that's not good for you—helps people soothe their blues away. When that food isn't there, they start panicking.

When you consciously make the decision that tomorrow will be a fast day, you activate a new mechanism inside yourself. You're forced to let your innards recharge while you reflect on the bad eating habits

# Sebastian's Story

Of all the suggestions in this book, it's likely the fast day that concerns you the most. Here's the thing: Choosing not to eat for an entire day often has some astonishingly pleasant results beyond losing weight. Consider Sebastian's story.

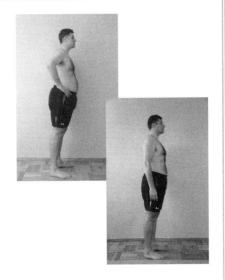

Deskbound at his job in New York City and superstressed day in and day out, he admits that he was an emotional eater, finding solace and satisfaction in all manner of junk. However, of all the things that helped him lose weight on this program—an astonishing 23 pounds—it's the fast day that he says helped him the most.

"Fasting was a revelation to me," says Sebastian. "I would never have thought that with all of the cravings I'd usually have, or with the dip that comes each afternoon that sends you running to the snack machine or for a coffee or pastry to sweeten your life. When you start doing the fast, you realize you can go for 18, 19, 20 hours without any food. Of course, you feel a little hungry, but it's not that uncomfortable, and it actually helps you get your mind focused."

Sebastian credits the 3-week time frame of the program, the tasty meals, and the plan's simplicity for his dramatic weight loss but remains wowed by the power of the fast day, a practice he plans to carry forward beyond his time on the plan.

"When breaking fast, I also profoundly realize that my body wants fresh food (salad, greens, fruit, berries) and is not attracted to greasy or sweet stuff. And that first food tastes so good!"

with which you've been self-medicating. Fasting is such a profound tool for deep change. No wonder people have been turning to it for centuries.

### 1-Day-Fast Food Guidelines

- On your fast days you will consume nothing but water or herbal tea. It's that simple.
- If you're taking any supplements (multivitamins, fish oil, etc.), give your body a break for a day.

### 1-Day-Fast Exercise Guidelines

- Take the day off and let your body work its magic.
- Or, engage in a longer-duration (1 hour or more) activity or very-low-intensity active recovery (walking, biking, etc.) that will rely on fat as its main fuel source.

## DAY 4: THE REGULAR-CALORIE DAY

Surprise, surprise: There's nothing special about this day. After the roller coaster of not eating carbs, eating nearly anything you like, then not eating at all, you're simply going to eat a regular diet today. That's it. The only rule, if you can call it that, is that you should do your best to eat real, whole foods.

### Regular-Cal Food Guidelines

The following Serving Size Simplifier should be used as a portion quantity guideline for each meal. Its intuitive approach is customized to your body size and will help you put calorie counting to rest for good. It was originally inspired by the amazing work done by my friends at Precision Nutrition.

- **Fibrous veggies:** 2 to 4 handfuls
- **Clean protein:** 1 palm-size portion for women, 1 to 2 palm-size portions for men

- **Starchy carbs and fruits:** 1 handful for women, 1 to 2 handfuls for men
- **Fit fats:** ½ shot glass (1½ tablespoons) for oils and butter (easier to measure/eyeball since these are generally poured); for nuts and seeds, 1 thumb-size serving for women, 2 thumb-size servings for men

Each element needs not be present at each meal, but do your best to keep them all in mind throughout the day. For instance, normally a green juice would consist of only leafy greens and other vegetables. However, you can power it up with a shot of flax oil or fish oil. Adding in these fats will not only stabilize your blood sugar but also improve your absorption of the fat-soluble vitamins found in the greens. With that said, I would strongly recommend that each time you eat (other than the odd apple here and there), you include protein and fiber in your meal. Doing so will prevent your blood sugar from rising and keep you full longer, both of which will help you lose fat instead of storing it.

For dinner, you might have a fillet of salmon (protein) cooked in butter (oil and fats) with a side of steamed greens (fibrous vegetables) and a small amount of quinoa (starchy carbs). Nuts and seeds would not be present in this meal—again, no big deal. You can always have a few almonds throughout the day. For solid meals (not smoothies or juices), these guidelines should yield a plate that is:

- One-half fibrous veggies
- One-quarter protein
- One-quarter starchy carbs (if applicable on that day) and oils and fats

Remember to listen to your body throughout the day so that you eat when you're hungry and stop when you're 80 percent full.

## What about Liquid Meals (Smoothies)?

When making a smoothie, these serving sizes still apply to the ingredients you put into your blender. For instance, one smoothie (that makes 2 to 3 servings) might include:

- 2 hand bowls of fibrous veggies → spinach, Swiss chard, etc.
- 1 palm-size portion of clean protein → a combination of almond butter, hemp seeds, and protein powder

## Antoinetta's Story

"Before the All-Day Fat-Burning Diet, I had gotten a bit out of control with my food choices and was feeling the consequences. In general, I always try to eat very natural, healthy foods (very little to no gluten, processed foods, sugar, etc.) but had gotten into a bad spell of eating a lot of junk. I was feeling 'blubbery' and ached with heartburn from stomach ulcers, which was starting to be a common occurrence again. (As a child, I had a lot of issues with getting sick every time I ate but doctors could never determine why. As an adult, I have finally figured out that I definitely have issues digesting foods that have artificial ingredients.)

"I thought that this program would be the perfect kick start to get me back on track and also to enhance my ability to really embrace and understand the choices I make day to day. And to be honest, Yuri's attitude of try-ing to seek improvement, not perfection, is 100 percent on par with how I approach my diet and how I want to teach the people around me to live. The all-or-nothing mentality that I feel a lot of health professionals promote is just too much for most people to handle—at least at Day 1 of their journey.

"After just 21 days, I am happy to say that I have not had one bit of heartburn or pain from my stomach ulcers since starting this program. I was worried about the fasting days because I thought there was no way that I could survive without severe stomach pain. Much to my surprise, never once did I have any pain. When I look in the mirror, I feel better about what I am seeing. My current measurements are down more than I expected—just the perfect boost to convince me that I am heading in the right direction."

- ½ to 1 handful of starchy carbs/fruit → 1 cup of berries
- ½ shot of fit fats → 1½ tablespoons flax oil or coconut oil

### *What about Green Juices?*

If you've followed my work, including my previous *New York Times* best-selling book *The All-Day Energy Diet*, you know that I'm a huge proponent of adding more fresh-pressed green juices into your diet. In my eyes, they are the magic bullet for achieving incredible energy and health. I'm not talking about the bottled, sugared-up "green" juices that you find at Starbucks or your local grocery store. I'm referring to fresh vegetable-based juices that you make from scratch at home.

When you make these, each version will have several handfuls of fibrous veggies but without their fiber, since juicing extracts the juice and discards the fiber. Thus, if you have a green juice, remember that all you are really getting is a ton of vital nutrients from fibrous veggies—no fiber, no clean protein, no starchy carbs, and no fit fats.

Starting your day with a green juice is great, but I would also suggest following your juice with something a little more substantial and balanced to keep you going longer. For instance, I'll often start my day with a green juice (when I'm not fasting or too lazy to make one) or drink a liter of water with my Energy Greens, and then about 30 to 60 minutes later I'll make some eggs or a protein shake or enjoy a protein-heavy cereal (like the "No Oat–Meal" on page 240).

## *Regular-Cal Exercise Guidelines*

Do a full-body workout—bodyweight, eccentric, or strength. (Don't worry, this will all be explained in the next chapter.)

# DAY 5: THE LOW-CALORIE DAY

You can consider this final 24 hours of your 5-day cycle a wind-down session. It's not as intense as a 1-Day Fast, but it is a gentle way for you to eat a little less than you did the day before. You accomplish this by simply eating about 25 percent less than you normally would.

## *Low-Cal Food Guidelines*

As usual, I'm not recommending that you count calories. Just reduce your portion sizes a little. The easiest way to hit the mark is to use the Serving Size Simplifier that I just mentioned. For example, just take a handful of starchy carbs but remove about one-quarter of that handful.

What you'll find in the meal plan for this program is that your

Low-Cal Days will tend to be filled with more raw foods and some lean proteins. The reason is that these foods are naturally lower in calories yet loaded with greater nutrients. You'll be able to eat as usual and still be under your regular caloric intake. That, in turn, will help your body shed some extra pounds.

You can also try any of the following:

- Use a slightly smaller plate, bowl, or cup than you normally would.
- Men: Use portion sizes based on a woman's hand size.
- Women: Use portion sizes based on a young teenager's hand size.

As with your Regular-Calorie Days and 1-Day Feasts, you want to focus on eating a well-balanced diet; don't restrict or eat an excessive amount of protein or fat. Simply follow the Serving Size Simplifier guidelines, take away about one-quarter from each serving, and that's it. Seriously, that's it!

## Low-Cal Exercise Guidelines

I'm sure you'll be delighted to hear this: Today is a day off. Use this day to let your body relax, recover, and bounce back. If you feel compelled to exercise, then just do some yoga or stretching, go for a walk, or do some very light cardio for no more than 15 to 20 minutes. Remember, a day off does not mean you should do nothing but sit on the couch. You still want to move throughout the day.

You should look forward to your days off because they are when your body has a chance to regenerate. Most people who love to exercise overdo it, thinking that more is better, but that belief leads to little more than overtraining injuries and stagnant results. Think about it this way: Your body repairs itself and grows during sleep. Would you ever deprive yourself of sleep? Not willingly. So think about your days off as being as necessary as sleep for your body. Don't rob it of the important downtime it needs to bounce back stronger. After all, tomorrow you'll start again.

Here's a quick overview of how the 5-Day Food-Cycling Formula will work over the next 21 days. And remember, there are *two* Low-

Carb Days to begin the plan so that we prime your body to rely more on fat than carbohydrates as its primary fuel source. I want you to get off to a great start!

| DAY 1 | DAY 2 | DAY 3 | DAY 4 | DAY 5 | DAY 6 | DAY 7 |
|-------|-------|-------|-------|-------|-------|-------|
| Low Carb | Low Carb | 1-Day Feast | 1-Day Fast | Regular Cal | Low Cal | Regular Cal |

| DAY 8 | DAY 9 | DAY 10 | DAY 11 | DAY 12 | DAY 13 | DAY 14 |
|-------|-------|--------|--------|--------|--------|--------|
| Low Carb | 1-Day Feast | 1-Day Fast | Regular Cal | Low Cal | Low Carb | 1-Day Feast |

| DAY 15 | DAY 16 | DAY 17 | DAY 18 | DAY 19 | DAY 20 | DAY 21 |
|--------|--------|--------|--------|--------|--------|--------|
| 1-Day Fast | Regular Cal | Low Cal | Low Carb | 1-Day Feast | 1-Day Fast | Regular Cal |

## CHAPTER 6

# STEP 4: EXERCISE USING THE "LIFT METHOD" TO BURN FAT 24/7

This is likely the chapter you've been dreading the most. Ironically, it's my favorite.

I never fail to be surprised by how much misunderstanding and trepidation surround working out. People who have not yet committed to a regular exercise routine have the general perception that you have to kill yourself to get in shape. Nothing could be further from the truth. In the 1970s, Jane Fonda popularized the phrase "No pain, no gain," and I wouldn't be surprised if that's where all these misconceptions started. What's sad is that this perspective keeps so many away from regular exercise; given how daunting it all seems, is it any surprise that people turn to diets instead? That's unfortunate, because diets alone are quite useless. That may sound like an overstatement, but it's not. We'll explore why shortly.

The truth is that regular exercise is essential to maintaining a trim and healthy physique. There is no way around it. However, spending hours on end running on a treadmill, doing situps, or bench-pressing extraordinarily heavy weights doesn't have to be part of the equation. In fact, it *never* should be. Make no mistake, exercise does take dedicated work on your part, but it doesn't require you to sacrifice all of your time and energy.

My clients are always stunned at just how little they have to exercise to achieve real and lasting results. That's the pleasant surprise I want you to experience. In this chapter, we're going to explore my unique LIFT method of exercise, which not only cuts down on the amount of time you spend exercising, but also guarantees substantial weight loss when performed in accordance with the eating and resting guidelines I've outlined in this program. In fact, it's my hope that you find yourself enjoying the routines I've created for you. Over the next 3 weeks, you'll find that good exercise doesn't drain you but, in fact, energizes you and gives you the charge you need to power through your days. What's more, you'll learn how simply staying active throughout the day through micromovements goes a long way toward keeping you slim. Sound too good to be true? It really isn't.

## WHY DIETS DON'T WORK AND EXERCISE DOES

I bet you've dieted before. If you haven't, someone close to you has. Either way, you're equipped to answer two questions for me: First, was it a pleasurable experience? Second, did it work?

The answer is likely no on both counts, right? I can't think of anyone I know who has honestly enjoyed dieting. It's always an ordeal people moan about, and all I can do is shake my head. What's more, even if they are successful in losing a few pounds, a few months later they find themselves right back where they started: chubby or overweight, complaining about how stressed and miserable they are, and trying to convince everyone—especially themselves—that they're going to start a new diet soon. I must say, it's tiring just thinking about it.

According to a January 2015 story in *U.S. News and World Report*, nearly two-thirds of dieters regain the weight they've lost on a diet within the first year.[1] That's a lot of people, especially when you consider that roughly 45 million Americans will try a new diet every year, according to figures from Boston Medical Center. That's a lot of time and energy being wasted, but the diet industry just keeps getting bigger and bigger. Those stats from BMC also reveal another surprising figure: Those 45 million people will collectively spend $33 billion each year on dieting methods.[2]

I am a part of that industry, but I'm positive my clients are in that small minority of dieters who drop their excess weight and keep it off. I'm telling you these statistics, though, because I don't want to mislead you, and I want you to know that I won't push any miracle pills or programs your way. I want to tell you the truth. That begins with telling you why dieting is pointless. Aside from the misery of it all, your body simply isn't programmed to respond to a diet in the way you've been told it will. Let me explain.

Your body is always using energy to perform all manner of external and internal functions, even when you're sleeping. This rate of energy use is called your *basal metabolic rate*. You gain energy from the food you eat in the form of calories, and this keeps your metabolic rate chugging along. If you eat more than you burn, your fat storage increases. Thus, the only way to make sure you're expending more energy than you're ingesting and storing is to increase your basal metabolic rate.

The only way to increase your basal metabolic rate is to increase your lean muscle, and the only way to increase your lean muscle is to exercise. It's really that simple.

This is precisely why diets don't work. When you diet, you deprive yourself of food and energy, and in the short term, this means that you lose weight. However, this also means that you gradually lower your basal metabolic rate. When you've achieved the weight-loss results you were aiming for and you start eating normally again, your food and energy intake will far exceed your lowered basal metabolic rate, and all the weight will start piling on again. It's an ugly and pointless cycle.

Thus, the only way to truly lose weight and keep it off is to take a multitiered approach: First, you have to incorporate healthier foods into your diet that promote hormonal balance and reduce inflammation inside your body. Second, you have to change your daily lifestyle to reduce stress and support positive growth. Finally, you have to exercise. That's right, you *have* to exercise.

Through exercise, you will gain lean muscle, which will increase your basal metabolic rate. With this increase, you will gradually become a fat-burning machine, even when you're not working out. Mind you, I'm not suggesting that you become a bodybuilder. That degree of pumped-up muscle isn't required to unlock the fat-burning properties of this program. I know this is especially a concern for women, most of whom want to avoid the muscled look. I assure you this is not what we're going for. I simply want you to be fit and firm.

Now this doesn't mean that you have to hit the gym 7 days a week. What I'm about to share with you flies in the face of convention. I think you'll find it to be a breath of fresh air. The key here is to make sure you're getting the right type and amount of exercise, and thankfully, utilizing the LIFT method is the perfect way to do both.

## THE LIFT METHOD

Let's get this out of the way: Despite the slick name, the LIFT method is not an exercise fad, technique, or tool like those you've seen advertised on cable television at 3:00 a.m. There are no 1-800 numbers to dial. There are no money-back guarantees. If anything, LIFT is a plan of attack. It stands for Length, Intensity, Frequency, and Tempo, as these are the parameters that we'll adjust to craft your ideal workout. Let's run them down, one by one.

### *Length*

This refers to the length of your workout. Depending on how overweight you are, you may be thinking that you have to put in hours of exercise to reach your goal weight. Well, you'll be pleased to hear that when it comes to exercise, more does not necessarily mean better. According to a study published in the January 2015 edition of the *Journal of the American College of Cardiology*, a moderate amount of exercise was proven to be more effective and even healthier than a large amount. In fact, excessive amounts of exercise were found to be potentially harmful![3]

The study—christened the Copenhagen City Heart Study—examined 1,098 healthy joggers and 3,950 healthy nonjoggers in Denmark over the course of 12 years. It found that those who ran more than 4 hours a week or more than 3 days a week turned out to have the same mortality risk as those who barely exercised. What's more, those who ran 1 to 2.4 hours a week and fewer than three times a week at a moderate pace had the lowest risk of dying!

This illustrates something that I've always told my clients: Too much working out is like driving your car into the ground. It's not sustainable, and over the long term, it's quite harmful. If you focus on the right type of exercise, then you don't have to perform it for hours on end. After all, who—other than professional athletes—has time for that? They're getting paid to exercise. We want to burn fat, so we need to spend less time working out. You'll be pleased to hear that, for our purposes, the sweet spot is less than 30 minutes. However, this brings us to the I in LIFT: If you're working out for a shorter period of time, your workout has to be of a higher intensity.

## Intensity

Make no mistake, if you want to lose weight, you will have to put in the work, and that means increasing the intensity of your workouts. There are different ways to accomplish this, the first being resistance training with weights, which requires you to engage and train your muscles more deeply than merely jogging or doing pushups would. In so doing, you will increase your basal metabolic rate, which accounts for 70 percent of the calories you burn every day.

I've prescribed the workouts you'll be performing in the guide later in this book, so try not to worry too much right now about how much weight you'll be lifting. All you need to know is that we're looking to hit the zone right between challenging and difficult. I want you to break a sweat when lifting these weights, but I don't want you to have a hernia.

The reassuring news is that because you'll be lifting challenging weights, you'll be doing a smaller number of repetitions—4 to 8 reps per round—to build muscle without the risk of becoming bulky or injuring yourself. We're aiming to hit exactly the right amount to get your metabolic rate pumped up.

When you lift challenging weights that require you to breathe in more oxygen (to fuel your working muscles), your body starts to pump out catecholamines, adrenal hormones that, among other things, trigger the breakdown of your fat stores. Countless studies show that spending less time doing higher-intensity work is the best way to burn fat and improve performance, whether that be your aerobic, anaerobic, or even strength performance.

The other method to increase the intensity of your workout is to incorporate as many full-body movements as possible. This engages more muscles in your body, which means your body needs more oxygen and so burns more calories. For example, instead of doing a simple biceps curl with a challenging weight, you can grab a weight from the floor, pick it up, curl it, then lift it above your head. This step-by-step movement is now activating far more than just your biceps, requiring you to use your leg muscles, core, and back and shoulder muscles.

Unlike many other plans, we're not going to focus on training muscle groups. We won't be doing a chest and arms day at the gym, followed by a legs day. As I said, we're not looking to turn you into anything even remotely resembling a bodybuilder, as this program is about losing fat, not gaining huge muscles. We're gunning for more well-rounded and intense workouts during this entire program that are then balanced with optimal recovery.

## Frequency

Frequency refers to how often you'll be working out, and on this program, that's three to four times a week. Some workout programs encourage you to get daily exercise, but given the intensity of our workouts, you'll need 24 to 48 hours of recovery time after each session. I can't overstate how important recovery time is to any exercise plan. Unfortunately, this important aspect of the process is commonly overlooked, but it's crucial when you're on a thorough plan. We want to avoid overtraining at all costs! I do, however, encourage you to remain active and walk every day for at least 30 minutes. This will also help with any soreness you might feel after your first few workouts.

### Tempo

Tempo is perhaps the most overlooked part of the LIFT method. It refers to the speed you use to lift weights during your session, and while it might not seem very important, it's essential to unlocking the muscle-building and fat-burning potential of each workout. The key here is to perform your movements properly and with the right focus. Good form is crucial, since by performing the movements correctly, you significantly diminish the likelihood of injury.

Here's how it works: You begin each lift explosively. By flexing your muscle to lift the weight in an explosive fashion, you're summoning as much strength (and thus muscle fibers) as possible and burning plenty of calories. The real magic, however, is in the next part of your lift—the lowering of the weight back to your starting position. Here, it's important to resist the pull of gravity by lowering the weight slowly, keeping your muscle engaged for as long as possible. Research shows that this is the phase of the lift—known as the *eccentric contraction*—where you get the strongest and burn the most fat. You're aiming for a very controlled descent of 4 to 6 seconds.

Remember: Most people sorely underestimate the importance of tempo when they hit the gym, but when incorporated into your workout with the other principles of the LIFT method, it becomes a very powerful tool.

## A DIFFERENT WAY TO DO CARDIO

The LIFT method applies to weight-lifting and even bodyweight exercises, but not to cardiovascular exercise, which is also an important part of your exercise schedule. That said, we're still going to do things a little differently than you may be used to. When you think of exercise, I'm sure the first thing that probably pops into your head is going to the gym and jumping on the treadmill to jog for an excruciating, extended period of time. There will be none of that here.

As we've seen, working out for extended periods of time can be harmful in the long term, and you can bet this applies to spending hours on end suffering on the treadmill. The same thing goes for long rowing sessions, long periods on the elliptical machines, or just about any type of cardio that requires you to set a steady pace and keep at it for an hour or more. What I'd like to suggest is that to burn more calories, more fuel, and ultimately more fat, it's important to train using intervals. For example, if you choose running as your form of cardio, rather than running or jogging for even 30 minutes straight, I'd like you to run for a bit, then jog for a bit, and repeat this cycle for the length of your workout. This is commonly known as *interval training*, and it has taken off over the last 10 years or so. And with good reason: Studies have routinely shown that this method is far more effective and healthier than long-form cardio.

Here's an analogy I like to make: As you know, driving in the city is far less fuel efficient than driving on the highway because you're constantly accelerating and braking. From a fuel perspective, this is less desirable than highway driving, as you're constantly paying more money to fill the gas tank. The exact opposite is true when you think about the car as your body and the fuel as fat. When you're constantly shifting between stopping and going, you kick in the same mechanism and burn more fuel. So intervals are the name of the game when it comes to fat loss, our very aim on this program. It's appropriate, then, that your workout week begin with interval training.

Now, let's look at which workouts you'll be doing in conjunction with the 5-Day Food-Cycling Formula to accelerate your fat loss and keep you lean for a long time to come.

# DAY 1: LOW CARB

## *Interval Speed Bursts*

On this day you're going to do just 5 to 10 minutes of sprint work. Don't worry, you won't be running alongside Usain Bolt on a 400-meter track (unless, of course, you want to pretend you are). The idea here is to use small amounts of high-intensity, burstlike activity to increase your body's release of catecholamines. These are your fight-or-flight hormones—specifically, epinephrine and norepinephrine—released by the adrenal glands in response to stress like high-intensity bursting. Yes, exercise is a form of stress. That's why we need to use it intelligently.

One of the roles of these stress hormones is to break down stored fat in your body into free fatty acids that can then be converted into energy. This intense exercise also depletes your glycogen stores much more readily. As glycogen is depleted, your body must rely further on burning fat for energy. You do not get this catecholamine response with low-intensity exercise. (If the word *intensity* scares you, don't be alarmed. You'll only be doing 5- to 10-second bouts interspersed with nice and easy recovery.)

You can do these interval speed bursts (aka interval training) on any cardio machine other than a treadmill. I know many people favor the treadmill, but it doesn't work here because it takes forever to change speeds. Here are a few ideas for interval speed bursts that get the job done.

- Sprinting on the beach or grass
- Sprinting on the stationary bike or elliptical
- Jumping rope
- Jumping jacks
- Running in place
- Running up and down stairs

Whichever exercise you choose, the key is to give it full-out, 100 percent effort. Again, don't let that scare you. You'll be fine. You won't have a heart attack. In fact, your heart will thank you because pushing out of your comfort zone is the only way to improve your aerobic capacity (aka max $VO_2$). A famous study published in the *Journal of Applied Physiology* in 2007 showed that just seven sessions of interval training increased the amount of fat burned in a subsequent, similar cycling session by 36 percent. Cardiovascular fitness also increased by

13 percent![4] Essentially, the female subjects of this study had become more efficient at relying on fat, instead of carbohydrates, as a major fuel source during exercise. Simply put, they became all-out fat burners!

Another study showed that as few as six sessions of high-intensity intervals over 2 weeks for a total of approximately 15 minutes of intense exercise increased skeletal muscle oxidative capacity and endurance performance and favored fat burning (instead of glycogen burning) during exercise.[5] Make no mistake, this is one of the key methods to activate all-day fat burning. Plus, since you'll be doing just a few minutes of intervals on a Low-Carb Day, your glycogen stores will already be more depleted than usual. This makes it both slightly more challenging and highly rewarding.

Here are three speed burst workout options to choose from based on your current fitness level.

### Interval Speed Burst #1: Beginner

5 seconds at 100 percent effort

20 seconds at recovery pace (nice and easy)

Repeat 10 times (about 4 minutes of total work)

### Interval Speed Burst #2: Intermediate

10 seconds at 100 percent effort

30 seconds at recovery pace

Repeat 5 times (just over 3 minutes of total work)

### Interval Speed Burst #3: Advanced

10 seconds at 100 percent effort

10 seconds at recovery pace

Repeat 15 times (5 minutes of total work)

If you'd like the "follow-along" versions of these workouts, go to my Web site, alldayfatburningdiet.com/resources.

Before you even attempt any of the above interval protocols, make sure you spend at least 5 minutes warming up your muscles to prevent injury and generate more bloodflow for the work ahead.

A good warmup should consist of the following:

- Aerobic component: 2 to 5 minutes of cardiovascular activity (jogging, cycling, skipping, etc.) that gradually increases in intensity. You should notice your body getting warm and even breaking a little bit of a sweat.

- Dynamic movement component: Now that your body is warm, it's time to work out the kinks, dust off the cobwebs, and get your muscles and joints used to the ranges of motion and movement patterns that you'll be encountering during the workout. At this stage, the goal isn't to stretch but rather to go through movements that will progressively loosen your muscles and lubricate your joints. Examples of dynamic warmup movements include lunge walks, inchworms, pushups, leg swings, and any other bodyweight movement that emphasizes flexibility, strength, and range of motion.

Your warmup should take about 5 to 7 minutes total and prepare you for the more intense activity you're about to undertake. Check out the following blog post for a great warmup: yurielkaim.com/1474 /dynamic-warm-up-exercises/.

## A CLEVER TRICK TO BURN MORE FAT

Pssst. I have a secret to share with you. It's a trick to help push your fat-burning capabilities further. Remember, immediately after you finish your speed bursts, free fatty acids (from broken-down fat) will flood into your bloodstream. Countless studies have shown that this is the time when your body, since it's recovering, really relies on those fats for fuel. For instance, a 2008 study showed that even though carbohydrates were the predominant fuel source during the actual workout, for more than 3 hours afterward, fats became the main contributor to energy.[6] Basically, the most fat was burned postworkout. But again, workout intensity sets the stage for this to happen.

Now, to really take advantage of this fat-burning window, I strongly recommend following your speed burst activity with 30 minutes (or more) of low-intensity cardio. This will help shuttle those free fatty acids floating around in your bloodstream into your muscles to be burned as fuel. Since I live in the Great White North, when it's warm outside, I'll go to the park and run sprints for a few minutes. Then, I'll simply go for a 30-minute walk with my dogs and kill two birds with one stone—walking the dogs and burning extra fat from exercise I would have done anyway. Or, if I'm traveling and happen to be close to the beach, I'll run sprints on the beach and follow up with a nice, long walk to discover the local area.

Remember, these low-intensity sessions are when your body prefers to use fat as its main fuel source—something most people don't understand. So make low-intensity activity work for you and pluck more of those low-hanging fruits (or, in this case, fats). The key is to keep moving so that your body uses the free fatty acids released from stored fat instead of being converted back into fat—a process known as *re-esterification*. It's really quite simple to make this work for you.

## SHOULD YOU EXERCISE ON AN EMPTY STOMACH?

For years, this has been one of the most common questions I've been asked by people looking to lose weight. In my mind, and according to a lot of the research I'm about to show you, it makes total sense to train in a fasted state on some workout days. I can tell you from first-hand experience that fasted high-intensity cardio like the interval speed bursts you'll be doing on Low-Carb Days produces superior fat-loss results.

Now, I know this goes against the golden rule of meal timing that I talked about earlier—that your biggest meal should come right after your workout—but on this one day, we're going to change things up and keep your body in a fasted state a little longer (1 to 2 hours) after you finish your short bout of sprints. I'll show you why in just a second.

But first, whenever you exercise in a fasted state, you must make sure of the following:

1. **Intensity is high.**
2. **Duration is short.**

In fact, intensity and duration are inversely related. After all, you can only sprint for so long, right? So it follows that if you're training for an hour, your intensity must be reduced to allow you to last that long. That's not what we want here. Remember, on your Low-Carb Days we're talking about 5 to 10 minutes of high-intensity work with the option of following those interval speed bursts with some light cardio for another 30 minutes or so.

Intensity is the key to losing fat and staying lean because it triggers the release of hormones that preserve muscle (i.e., growth hormone and testosterone) and help unlock stored fat (i.e., epinephrine). If possible, do your best to perform your interval speed bursts (and most of your workouts in this program) first thing upon waking in the morning after an overnight fast. If your schedule only allows you to work out later in the evening, make sure to wait 3 to 4 hours after a meal before training for maximum fat burning. This will ensure that insulin is low and your body more readily taps into its fat stores as a source of fuel for your workout.

Research has suggested that carb intake before or during an exercise session can blunt the expression of several metabolic genes following exercise. Insulin may play a role here.[7] Another way to think of it is that providing nutrients to the body makes it experience exercise as less of a stressor than fasted-state training. Why should it adapt or compensate when all the fuel it needs has been provided?

So should you exercise in a fasted state all the time? I don't think so. But you certainly can on certain days, like your Low-Carb Days, when carb intake (and thus insulin) will be low anyway. Or you can simply listen to your body and, if it's okay with training in a fasted state, go for it. You'll burn more fat as a result. I wouldn't recommend this approach for athletes or those looking to pack on pounds of muscle, but again, that's not the focus of this program. We're here to burn fat and turn your body into a 24/7 fat-burning machine.

Fasted exercise means that you're working out when your blood sugar and glycogen stores might be a little low. This often makes fasted workouts more challenging—you simply don't have enough fuel in the tank. But again, we're exercising at a high intensity for only 5 to 10 minutes here, so you should be fine.

In general, I do suggest that the great majority of your daily allotment of calories and carbs be ingested in the postworkout period, not before. If you must eat before you train, the immediate preworkout meal should contain very few low–glycemic index carbs. And if it's a Low-Carb Day, you're exercising for only 5 to 10 minutes, in which case your body already has plenty of glycogen fuel to draw on.

You don't have to do all of your workouts for the rest of your life in a fasted state, but at least for these 21 days, I recommend that you do your Low-Carb Day interval speed bursts that way. The cool part about fasted exercise and higher-intensity exercise is that both train your body to become a better fat-burning machine. And they've even been shown to have favorable effects on muscle building compared with training in a fed state, especially where strength training has been employed. This can be very helpful to keep in mind on your 1-Day Feast and Regular-Cal training days, so I'll go into more detail about it in those sections.

If you absolutely must have something to eat before this short workout, then have a small amount of protein (such as protein powder in water) because of its beneficial effect on your metabolic rate.

To summarize:

- Ideally, do your interval speed bursts on an empty stomach to keep insulin levels low and to allow your body to rely more heavily on fat.

- Alternatively, ingest 30 grams of protein 10 to 15 minutes before exercising.

- Break your fast postworkout. Your biggest meal should come within 1 hour of your workouts except on your Low-Carb Days, when I challenge you to stay in a fasted state for 1 to 2 hours postworkout.

- If you have blood sugar issues and feel you need to eat something right after your workout, then please do so. That's better than passing out, right? As always, consult your doctor.

## WHAT TO EAT AFTER YOUR WORKOUT

I believe your most important meal of the day is your postworkout meal. After a workout is when your muscles are ready to soak up carbs to refuel and protein to rebuild, as well as other vital nutrients. However, I'm making an exception on your Low-Carb Days because, after your interval speed bursts, you can maximize your reliance on fat postworkout (without compromising your lean muscle mass) by not eating anything for a little while longer.

We've seen that high-intensity exercise forces your body to release all kinds of fat-burning hormones by ramping up your sympathetic nervous system. This is what helps create a fat-burning hormonal environment inside your body. However, the minute you consume calories, you'll spike your body's primary storage hormone—insulin. Again, this is totally fine on most days, when we want our biggest meal right after our workout.

The beauty of occasionally not eating right after a workout (at least on your Low-Carb Days) is that the absence of insulin and presence of adrenaline set the stage for a heavier reliance on fat breakdown instead of fuel storage. The other amazing part of a short fast postworkout is that the body actually releases more growth hormone (GH) as a way of preserving lean muscle tissue.

Fasting and intense exercise are two of the only natural ways (in addition to deep sleep) to increase GH. And that's very important for preserving your muscle mass, which keeps your metabolic rate highly active and churning through fat all day long.

Your body knows what it needs to do to survive. In a short-term fasted state, your body will go to great lengths to preserve its muscle. And the more muscle you maintain, the healthier your metabolic rate and the more fat you burn. This is contrary to the old-school advice that not eating will put you into fat-storing survival mode, deplete your muscle, and ruin your metabolism.

# DAY 2: THE 1-DAY FEAST
## *Full-Body Metabolic Conditioning*

The only thing as damaging to our waistlines as the popularity of the low-fat movement of the 1980s was the "cardio is better for weight loss" movement that gained popularity during the same time. What a mess it has caused.

As you'll see in this program, the only cardio I'm recommending is your 5 to 10 minutes of interval speed bursts and the occasional 30-minute light cardio session when you're in a fasted state. Walking on a daily basis should be a given. Other than that, we're going to stop wasting hours upon hours slaving over cardio machines.

In the last decade, a lot of research has revealed that long, slow cardio workouts can actually sabotage your ability to burn fat. Think about that for a moment. If you're tired, fed up, and disappointed with the results you've been getting from your current workout, then I want you to know that this cutting-edge research is going to change your life. You'll also see exactly how the entire fitness industry—from personal trainers to gym owners to equipment manufacturers—has it all wrong when it comes to losing fat.

The good news is that the tide is slowly shifting. If you've been told that you need to do up to an hour of cardio per day to lose weight, then you should know that's a big fat lie. Remember, exercise—especially when done improperly (like doing too much cardio)—is a big stress on your body. It puts your body into survival mode, in which it switches to its "store and hold on to fat" setting. Other studies show that excessive cardio can not only make you fatter, but accelerate the aging process.

The truth is that when you switch from relying on cardio to doing the unique, short-burst workouts in the All-Day Fat-Burning Diet, you'll shed fat quicker and feel better in just a few weeks. I'm tired of seeing well-intentioned people waste their time in the gym. I don't want you to feel stuck. I don't want you to hate your body and feel ashamed of the way you look. Most people believe that the key to losing fat and getting in shape is to spend lots of time running on a

## Ellen's Story

Something really important happens when you commit to this plan: You learn so much about yourself. Whether it's your reaction to a fast or insight into your terrible food choices, there's simply no way you can come away from this experience without understanding yourself better. Ellen is a perfect example.

About a year before she started this program, Ellen began working with a naturopathic doctor who helped her tackle her weight issues. "Multiple doctors over the years had just kept telling me to eat less, exercise more, and eat less salt," says Ellen. "I knew that was not my problem but couldn't get anyone to listen."

This doctor was different, however, and by ridding her diet of many of the foods we list here as our enemies, she lost more than 60 pounds. As great as that was, Ellen still wasn't feeling quite right. She wanted to go further.

Over the course of 6 weeks on this program, Ellen lost 10 more pounds, but more importantly, she was able to get a new handle on herself.

"What Yuri has provided me is control of my eating where I don't have to crave so much, and I also don't have to feel guilty if I don't eat so much," shares Ellen. "Being able to feel like I have control of my body is a wonderful change! I still have a few more pounds to go. I see this as a journey and look forward to learning more about what works best for me, my body, and my lifestyle."

treadmill. And as a former pro soccer player who's seen firsthand what too much running can do to your body, I can tell you that excessive cardio is a ticking time bomb waiting to go off. You see, long-duration cardio actually trains your body to store fat. It makes your body *guard* its fat. Why? Because of what it does to your hormones.

We've seen many times already in this book that your hormones are largely responsible for whether or not your body is a fat burner or a fat storer. According to a study in the *European Journal of Applied Physiology*, 20 weeks of daily cardio among women led to significant decreases in T3 (that vital thyroid hormone that controls your metabolism) and leptin (the "I'm full" hormone). The researchers speculated that these unfavorable hormonal drops were a means of energy conservation in these exercising women.[8]

Why would they need to conserve energy? Because their bodies were stressed by the sheer amount of exercise. And what happens when your body undergoes prolonged stress? It switches to fat-storing mode. It slows down your metabolism as a way of conserving energy, which means you won't be burning fat. But it gets worse. Prolonged endurance training, particularly running, is linked with protein loss from muscle partially induced by cortisol and lowered testosterone levels.[9] Less muscle means a lower metabolic rate, which means fewer calories burned. Plus, those who consistently do cardio endurance training typically have a higher cortisol response.

Cortisol is associated with heart disease, cancer, and visceral belly fat. That's the kind of fat that hangs around your waist—nobody wants that. I should note that the short, intense workouts in this program also increase cortisol, but to nowhere near the same degree as do high-volume, long-duration cardio workouts. Again, it is important to distinguish between acute (short-term) and chronic (long-term) cortisol release. When muscle glycogen concentrations run low, cortisol is released and fuel use shifts toward fat so that judicious use is made of the little glucose (sugar) that remains. However, in the long term, with too much cardio, excessive cortisol will encourage fat synthesis and storage and even age you faster.

Doing too much cardio is similar to constantly being stressed out. Eventually, you'll pay the price. So let me ask you a question: How many professional athletes do you see playing past 35 years of age? Not many, right? You could probably count them on one hand. And those who have managed to make it past 35 probably look 5 to 7 years older than they really are. The reason is simple—it's a question of wear and tear. Too much and the wrong type of exercise wear you down and will age you faster than a grape sitting in the sun.

An article in the *Journal of Strength and Conditioning Research* found that cardio causes immense oxidative damage and a flood of free radicals in the body.[10] Free radicals are molecules that cause rapid aging in your body. During long cardio sessions, your body is filled with free radicals that float around in your bloodstream and attack your cells like street thugs. Not only do free radicals cause damage to all your organs, but doing cardio also damages your skin and makes you look older. That's why many hard-core runners and older pro athletes look like 60-year-old sun worshippers. That might be a bit of a stretch (no pun intended), but you get the idea. They look and feel older than they are. You don't want that, do you?

Now, if high cortisol, low T3, and accelerated aging weren't bad enough, endurance cardio training also increases your appetite. In fact, your body reacts to cardio like a dramatic teenager to the word *no*, making you do exactly what's bad for you—eat more and more food. Even worse, you always end up eating more fat-promoting calories *after* you work out, which means that you gain more and more weight. A 2008 study in the *International Journal of Obesity* found that after cardio exercise, the subjects ate 100 calories more than they had just burned off in their workout. The researchers found that even reading had less of a calorie rebound effect than these workouts.[11]

I hope you're starting to realize that too much cardio is really a big waste of time and sets you up for fat-loss failure in the long run by disrupting your precious hormone balance and sabotaging your body.

## When Is More Not Better?

Cardio is not the only problem. Too much of any kind of exercise is just as bad. The trouble is that nowadays we're surrounded by infomercials and exercise programs that have you working out like a navy SEAL six or seven times per week. No wonder the very mention of the word *exercise* is so terrifying! Sure, you'll see visible results from doing such work, but you're also laying the foundation for severe problems down the road.

Exercise is a form of stress, so more is not better. Too much training has been shown to have harmful effects on the immune system.

Research has shown that the cellular damage that occurs during over-training can lead to nonspecific, general activation of the immune system, including changes in natural killer cell activity and the increased activation of peripheral blood lymphocytes. This hyperactivity of the immune system following intense overtraining may possibly even contribute to the development of autoimmune conditions.

Earlier we discussed how using short, interval-like exercise is terrific for burning fat. But as with anything, the poison is in the dosage. One study had men go through two intensive interval-training sessions per day for 10 days, followed by 5 days of active recovery. Not surprisingly, these men became acutely overtrained, as indicated by significant reductions in running performance from day 1 to day 11, severe fatigue, immune system deficits, mood disturbances, physical complaints, sleep difficulties, and reduced appetite.[12]

I often tell my clients that there's a lot to learn from the extremes. My experience as a pro soccer player and collegiate strength and conditioning coach has given me some unique perspectives about training intelligently, whether the goal is improved performance or fat loss. Let's look at the case of marathon runners—perhaps the best example of how too much training can harm your body. Countless studies have shown that marathoners, although touted for their athletic prowess, are actually very unhealthy. I can relate. As an extremely active teenager, I was fit but very unhealthy. And ignoring that fact led me to develop an autoimmune condition.

It's been shown that marathoners are at an increased risk of developing upper respiratory tract infections following races and periods of hard training, which are associated with changes in the immune system. Furthermore, it has been hypothesized that during this period of immune suppression, viruses and bacteria can gain a foothold, which can increase the risk of infections.[13] The two elements that may have been destroying your body and sabotaging your fat loss—long cardio training and too much intense training of any kind—are not present in the All-Day Fat-Burning Diet. The goal of this program is to reset your metabolism, improve your hormonal function, and help your body regain its fat-burning capabilities. For that reason, we eat and train in ways that are smarter and less stressful on the body.

**"Okay, Yuri, if cardio and too much exercise are so bad for me, what should I do instead?"**

I'm glad you asked. Right now I'm going to show you exactly what you should be doing instead of cardio and daily workouts that run your body into the ground. The workout plan I've laid out for you in this program has been used for years by thousands of my clients and produces astonishing body transformations without fail. The best part is that you'll be working out for only 90 minutes *per week* to get an amazing body.

Let me put that into perspective for you. Ninety minutes is:

- The duration of one soccer game
- The average length of a movie
- The length of a flight from Toronto to New York City

And none of those activities is setting you up for the body you deserve. So let's be honest—you can do this. You can find time just three times per week to make smart exercise a priority for you. Note that I didn't say "squeeze in a workout" because the truth is that your workouts should be scheduled into your calendar like anything else that's important in your life.

The workouts you're going to perform in this program involve the LIFT method that I described earlier and are fundamental to keeping you lean and strong. We've discussed the importance of exercise intensity—when used properly—for burning fat. And we've seen that spending all your time slugging away on the cardio machines—although better than doing nothing—is really wasting your time because it makes your body hold on to fat and break down more quickly. The best part of the All-Day Fat-Burning Diet workouts is that instead of doing an hour of weights and then spending an hour on the cardio machines, you'll get greater results by merging both into a shorter, more intense workout. You'll end up spending about one-third the training time but getting *double* the results.

If it sounds like I'm selling you snake oil, let me reassure you that this method of training has been proven to be more effective than just about any other workout method out there. The science speaks for itself. One study looked at obese premenopausal women to figure out whether traditional steady-state cardio was as effective as what I'm describing for burning fat. Each group exercised three times per week for 8 weeks and expended 300 calories per exercise session. Max $VO_2$, body composition, and resting metabolic rate were measured before and after training.

Not surprisingly, both max $VO_2$ and body composition did not improve in the steady-state cardio group but improved significantly in the higher-intensity exercise group. Plus, resting metabolic rate remained elevated in the latter for an additional 24 hours, meaning that more fat was burned for an entire day after the workout was over![14] For some reason, resistance training has often been overlooked by the many men and women who want to burn fat. But it shouldn't be because it's arguably the most important element in getting that strong, lean look. Even folks who do resistance training traditionally see it as separate from cardio. That means they end up spending more time working out to address both components. I don't know about you, but I don't have all day to be doing hours of both cardio and resistance training. Thankfully, you won't have to with this program.

Not only is resistance training critical for building strong bones and preventing osteoporosis—especially for women—but it's really the only way to ensure that you build and preserve your lean muscle, the driving force behind your metabolic rate. I like to think of resistance training as a long-term investment in your body. As you stimulate, build, and pre- serve your muscle tissue by working against resistance (bodyweight or weights), you set up your body to burn fat 24/7 for a long time to come. Long-duration cardio, on the other hand, is a short-term investment at best since it has zero positive impact on preserving your lean muscle mass in the long run. In fact, it actually breaks it down, which sends your metabolic rate plummeting.

One of the reasons many people gain weight as they age is the slow- ing of their metabolic rate. Since muscle is the most metabolically active (i.e., calorie-churning) component of your body, losing it slows your metabolism and increases your chances of gaining weight. This naturally occurs in all humans, as we begin to lose muscle mass on a yearly basis starting at about 30 years old. So keeping muscle is imperative to get the body you want. The All-Day Fat-Burning Diet workouts address the limitations of traditional exercise protocols and provide more effective fat burning while saving you a lot of time. These resistance-training programs come in two flavors, and I recommend that you use them on specific days of the 5-day caloric-cycling plan. I call them *full-body metabolic conditioning (FBMC)* and *eccentric strength workouts.*

## Full-Body Metabolic Conditioning (FBMC) Workouts

Here, resistance-training exercises (using both bodyweight and weights) are structured in a way that challenges your muscles while eliciting a great cardiovascular workout. These workouts will make you huff and puff and get you sweating—two hallmark features of a high-intensity workout that will burn calories both during and after your workout. Over the past 15 years, I've developed thousands of FBMC programs. The number of ways to structure these workouts is truly endless.

In this program, you'll benefit from the fat-burning magic of my famous *minicircuits,* in which you'll perform three full-body exercises back-to-back with limited rest (anywhere from 15 to 30 seconds). You'll repeat this three-exercise minicircuit, then follow it up with interval speed bursts. Next, you'll tackle a new three-exercise minicircuit, also performing it twice and following it with a set of interval speed bursts. This workout strengthens and tones all the major muscles in your body and gets your heart rate pumping (great for cardiovascular health) in less than 30 minutes.

A ton of research has shown that this type of intense training, using full-body exercises known to significantly elevate your heart rate along with minimal rest periods, provides maximum fat burning in very little time.[15, 16, 17] Why do these FBMC workouts burn fat so well?

First, resistance training, which challenges your muscles, contributes significantly to the amount of fat burned during a workout.[18] Second, when resistance-training exercises using multiple large muscles are combined with very little rest between sets, they elicit aerobic and metabolic benefits that last for hours postworkout—a concept known as EPOC (which I'll describe shortly).[19, 20] Additionally, the higher intensity of these workouts increases the level of fat-burning catecholamines such as epinephrine and muscle-preserving growth hormone found in the blood both during and after your workout.[21, 22] And, with limited time to recover, shorter rest periods force your muscles to demand more oxygen, which leads to a higher heart rate (to deliver that oxygen). All of these factors contribute to burning more calories.

Since these workouts require effort and energy, you'll be performing them during your well-fueled 1-Day Feasts. These higher-carb, higher-calorie days set the stage for a higher-intensity full-body workout. For maximum fat loss, it's best to do these workouts *before* your biggest meal of the day.

### The Afterburn: Passive Fat Loss

Above, I briefly alluded to something called EPOC. This stands for "excess postexercise oxygen consumption." It represents the increased rate of oxygen intake following strenuous activity, which is needed to make up for the "oxygen deficit" created during the workout. It should be noted that EPOC is virtually nonexistent after slow cardio workouts but very elevated after interval training and bouts of higher-intensity exercise. In a nutshell, the higher the intensity, the longer the EPOC.

You can think of EPOC as the "afterburn" of a challenging workout. Earlier, I mentioned that resistance-training workouts are the ultimate long-term investment in a lean body. Well, when structured in an FBMC model, they also become an amazing short-term investment by burning calories not only during the workout but, in some cases, up to 72 hours after it's completed.[23] Imagine doing one FBMC workout and having your metabolic rate remain elevated and churning through fat calories for up to 3 days. That's incredible! That's what I call passive fat loss. You will literally be burning calories while watching TV or working at the office. Think about it like this: If you do an FBMC workout on a Monday, you'll burn extra fat all day Tuesday and into early Wednesday morning—and all because you trained smarter, not longer.

This is precisely why you only need to work out 3 days per week to get great results. You'll train your body to burn fat on the 4 days you're not working out, so you need to exercise for only 90 minutes to burn fat 24 hours per day, 7 days per week. Using our investment model, you make a quick 30-minute workout investment that sets you up in the long run for a strong, lean body, while also providing immediate and passive fat-loss returns for hours or days after your initial investment. Pretty cool, right?

Here's an example of a beginner Full-Body Metabolic Conditioning workout. For more advanced options and audio and video versions to exercise along with, go to alldayfatburningdiet.com/resources.

## Full-Body Metabolic Conditioning Workout: Beginner

### Protocol

2 tri-sets + 1 minute of speed bursts x 2 sets

### Tri-Set #1 (rest up to 30 seconds between exercises)

Dumbbell Sumo Squats x 6 reps (20 seconds)

Single-Arm Back Rows x 6 reps/side (40 seconds)

Kettlebell Swings x 6 (20 seconds)

### Complete two sets, then do interval speed bursts as follows:

5 seconds @ 100 percent

20 seconds of recovery

Repeat 4 times.

**Rest 2 minutes, and move to:**

**Tri-Set #2 (limit rest to 30 seconds between exercises)**

Stepups x 6 reps/leg (40 seconds)

Dumbbell Chest Presses x 6 reps (20 seconds)

Lat Pulldowns x 6 reps (20 seconds)

**Complete two sets, then do interval speed bursts as follows:**

5 seconds @ 100 percent

20 seconds of recovery

Repeat 4 times.

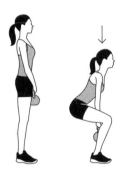

# DUMBBELL SUMO SQUATS

**Muscles worked: legs**

Stand with your feet 4 to 6 inches wider than your shoulders, with your toes pointed out at a 45-degree angle. Hold a dumbbell with both hands in the center of your body. While keeping your back straight, descend slowly by bending at the knees and hips as if you are sitting down into a chair. Lower yourself until your thighs are parallel to the floor. Return to the starting position by pressing upward and extending your legs while maintaining an equal distribution of weight on your forefoot and heel. Repeat for the prescribed number of repetitions.

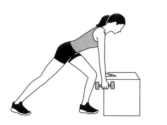
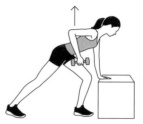

# SINGLE-ARM BACK ROWS

**Muscles worked: back, biceps**

Choose a flat bench and place a dumbbell on each side of it. Move your right leg back, bend your torso forward from the waist until your upper body is at a 45-degree angle to the floor, and place your left hand on the other end of the bench for support. Use your right hand to pick up the dumbbell on the floor and hold the weight while keeping your lower back straight. The palm of your hand should be facing your torso.

Pull the weight straight up to the side of your chest, keeping your upper arm close to your side and keeping your torso still. Focus on squeezing your back muscles so that your shoulder blade moves inward toward your spine. Lower the weight straight down toward the floor and repeat for the specified amount of repetitions. Switch sides and repeat with the other arm.

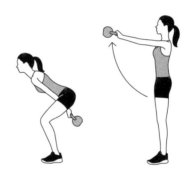

# KETTLEBELL SWINGS

**Muscles worked: glutes, hamstrings, lower back, core**

Stand with your feet slightly wider than shoulder-width apart, toes pointed out, and knees slightly bent; look straight ahead. Hold the kettlebell with both hands using a two-handed, overhand grip just in front of your hips.

Keeping your core strong and back flat, bend your hips back until the kettlebell is between and behind your legs; squeeze your glutes to extend your hips and swing the weight up. Let the weight swing back between your legs as you bend your hips and slightly bend your knees. Extend your hips and knees to reverse the momentum as you immediately begin the next rep.

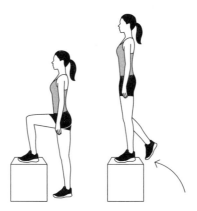

# STEPUPS

**Muscles worked: legs**

Find a step, chair, or bench that when you place your foot on it, your knee bends to a 90-degree angle. Place your entire left foot onto the bench or chair. Press through your left heel as you step onto the bench, bringing your right foot to meet your left so you are standing on the bench. Return to the starting position by stepping down with the left foot, then the right so both feet are on the floor. Perform for the required number of reps.

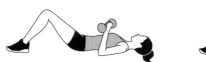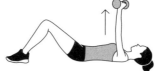

# DUMBBELL CHEST PRESSES

**Muscles worked: chest, shoulders, triceps**

Lie down on the floor or a flat bench with a dumbbell in each hand resting just outside each shoulder. The palms of your hands will be facing each other. Then, using your thighs to help raise the dumbbells up, lift the dumbbells one at a time so that you can hold them in front of you at shoulder width as you lie back onto the bench. The dumbbells should be just to the sides of your chest, with your upper arm and forearm creating a 90-degree angle. Then, push the dumbbells up and slightly to the middle. Lock your arms at the top of the lift and squeeze your chest, hold for a second, and then begin coming down slowly. Repeat for the required number of reps.

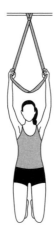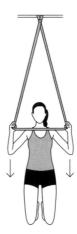

# LAT PULLDOWNS

**Muscles worked: back, biceps, forearms**

Sit down on a pull-down machine with a wide bar or band attached to the top pulley. Make sure that you adjust the knee pad of the machine to fit your height. These pads will prevent your body from being raised by the resistance attached to the bar.

Grab the bar with your palms facing forward about 1 foot wider than your shoulder on each side. Recline your torso back slightly (about 30 degrees), then bring the bar down until it touches your upper chest by drawing your shoulders and upper arms down and back. Concentrate on squeezing your back muscles once you reach the full contracted position. Your upper torso should remain stationary and only your arms should move. Return by slowly raising the bar back to the starting position so your arms are fully extended and your lats are fully stretched. Repeat this motion for the prescribed amount of repetitions.

# DAY 3: 1-DAY FAST

## Rest or Active Recovery

Your 1-Day Fast is an opportunity to give your body a much-needed break from constant digestion so it can relax and repair. Plus, since you won't be eating or drinking anything on this day other than water or herbal tea, you won't necessarily have the energy to go through an intense workout. That's why on this day you should focus on rest, relaxation, and recovery. As always, you can go for a nice walk since daily movement is important. Be sure to drink plenty of water during your fast so that your body is well hydrated to flush out built-up toxins and acids. And if you have a foam roller, spend some time rolling out your muscles—it's like having your own personal massage therapist.

# DAY 4: REGULAR CAL

## Eccentric Strength and Bodyweight Workouts

On your Regular-Cal Days, you can choose to do an eccentric strength, bodyweight, or bodyweight eccentrics workout, depending on your fitness level and training goals. Bodyweight might be a great place to start if you're not used to working out. However, even for more advanced exercisers like myself, bodyweight workouts can still be challenging. Whichever type of workout you choose, be sure to start with a good warmup and even a quick run-through set in which you perform 2 or 3 reps of each exercise (with lighter weights if it's a strength workout).

### Eccentric Strength Workouts

To provide a different stimulus to your body and foster the development of muscular strength (not necessarily size) while saving you tons of workout time, try one of my *eccentric strength* workouts. I offer them in two flavors, one using bodyweight and one using weights. Whichever you choose, you will benefit from the muscle- and strength-building power of what I call explosive-slow training. For instance, instead of doing as many pushups as you can as quickly as you can, eccentric training focuses on pushing explosively and lowering slowly.

Eccentric training is defined as active contraction of a muscle while the muscle is lengthening. For example, in a biceps curl, the action of lowering the dumbbell back down from the lift is the eccentric (aka "negative") phase of that exercise. Here, the biceps are in a state of contraction to control the rate of descent of the dumbbell. The eccentric phase is also what causes delayed onset muscle soreness (DOMS) about 48 hours after a workout. But don't worry, that soreness won't happen each time you train—just the first few times, until your body has adapted. For instance, completing bouts of eccentric training and then repeating the workout 1 week (or more) later will result in less DOMS after the second workout.[24]

Eccentric training provides a multitude of benefits to the human body, including the following:

- Protection from injury or reinjury
- Less weariness (feeling of extreme fatigue) from training
- Potential to raise resting metabolic rate by about 9 percent, with the greatest magnitude in the first 2 hours[25]
- Greater strength and performance improvements[26]

Eccentric strength workouts, where lowering weights *slowly* is the focus, improve strength and fat loss since safely lifting and slowly lowering heavy things enables us to generate more force. And here's the best part about eccentric strength workouts: You don't need to do them very often, nor do you need to follow the typical old-school recommendation of three sets of 10 to 12 repetitions in order to see significant strength and metabolic improvements.

An illuminating review of the research more than 15 years ago, which for some reason still hasn't caught on with mainstream fitness gurus, revealed that for training durations of 4 to 25 weeks, there is no significant difference in the increase in strength as a result of training with single versus multiple sets.[27]

In our eccentric strength workouts, you'll benefit from both time-saving one-set workouts and arguably more effective (for strength gains) two-set protocols. Furthermore, since you'll be putting your muscles under greater stress (in a good way) but lifting heavier weights at a slower tempo, you won't need to work out as often as you might think. A 2007 study compared strength differences between two groups of untrained women who performed a single set (6 to 10 repetitions to muscular failure) of the leg press exercise either once or twice per week. After 8 weeks, researchers found that performing a single set of the leg press once or twice per week resulted in statistically similar strength gains in these untrained women.[28]

The challenge is that we tend to think that if a little is great, then more must be better. But remember, we want you to get great results without spending all your time in the gym. Even if you have a lot of time to work out, I still recommend that you train smarter, not longer.

When I was studying at the University of Toronto, I would often observe how sprinters trained. It was quite odd. I noticed that these sprinters spent half their workouts talking on the phone or chatting with friends. That couldn't be right, could it? Weren't they wasting their time? Yet, something they were doing worked because these men and women were true specimens—lean, muscular, and healthy looking.

From a fat-loss perspective, it certainly wouldn't help you to work out like this, but then I realized that these sprinters were in the game of developing strength and power. Therefore, they required ample rest between explosive bouts. They would sprint 50 meters and then chill out for a few minutes. Then they'd go again. Same in the weight room—they would perform an explosive Olympic lift for 2 or 3 reps, and then take what seemed like an eternity of rest between sets. That's kind of the idea with our eccentric strength workouts. Although you won't have 5 to 10 minutes of rest between sets, the goal is to focus on giving 100 percent effort in each exercise. As a result, you won't need to do three or four sets or need to work out four or five times per week.

These eccentric strength workouts will differ from the FBMC workouts in a number of ways.

1. **You will have more recovery time between exercises.** Since the goal is strength and lean muscle gains, you don't need to be huffing and puffing or sweating up a storm. With a little more rest between exercises, you'll have the energy necessary to perform each subsequent repetition to the best of your ability.

2. **You will perform very few repetitions, 4 to 8 on average.** Once again, our goal in this program is not to build pounds of muscle but rather to develop a strong, lean body. You don't achieve that by swinging around 5-pound dumbbells for 20 reps. One study divided untrained subjects into four groups: a low-repetition group performing 3 to 5 reps maximum (RM) with 3 minutes of rest between sets and exercises, an intermediate-repetition group performing 9 to 11 RM with 2 minutes of rest, a high-repetition group performing 20 to 28 RM with 1 minute of rest, and a nonexercising control group. Not surprisingly, the low-repetition group had the greatest strength gains. The important thing to remember is that when strength and low reps are the goal, you should be lifting a heavy enough weight that you can do only the number of reps required. If you can perform more reps, then you're lifting too light a weight for the purpose of strength improvements.

3. **You will use heavier weights (except, of course, for the bodyweight exercises).** This is your chance to make significant strength gains and increase your metabolic rate as a result, no matter your age or fitness level. A study in the *Journal of Applied Physiology* looked at whether heavier-weight strength training over 16 weeks could increase strength and metabolic rate among 50- to 65-year-old men. Of course it did! Average strength levels increased 40 percent, body fat decreased, and resting metabolic rate increased by 7.7 percent.[29] You don't get these results by lifting light weights. And if you're using only the weight of your body, the "explosive-slow" tempo will ensure that each rep is a suitable challenge for you.

4. **You will use an "explosive-slow" tempo.** An example is a 1-second explosive push or pull, no pause at the top of the movement, and a 5- to 6-second slow return to the starting position. Moving resistance in an explosive, yet controlled, manner recruits more muscle fibers, which means you'll burn more calories and develop greater

strength. One study proved this very point by revealing that subjects who did the lifting (concentric) phase of biceps curls faster over an 8-week period showed greater strength improvements than those doing slower-speed lifts.[30] Even if the weight (or your body) doesn't move quickly, your intention should be to push or pull it quickly, then return slowly to the starting position.

## Another Reason Traditional Cardio Sucks

Just when you thought I was done talking about the downside of cardio, I'm back for more.

We just looked at the benefits of lifting (and lowering) heavier weights and moving that weight explosively in the concentric portion and slowly in the eccentric portion. Another reason for doing this is that you train different muscle fibers in the process.

Most people think steady-state exercise is good because it gets a lot of muscles involved. But the reality is that long, slow exercise activates only one of the four types of muscle fibers we have. Doing more of it simply works that one type of muscle fiber over and over. Sadly, that single type of muscle fiber is the least effective at triggering the hormonal reaction required to most efficiently burn body fat while preserving lean tissue. That's why cross-country and long-distance athletes look like they've spent most of their lives on *Survivor*, while sprinters (who tap into the other three types of muscle fiber) are strong and lean.

To dig a bit deeper, it's helpful to understand how our muscles function.

- We have different types of muscle fibers that do different things; for instance, slow-twitch fibers for long, slow activity and fast-twitch fibers for short-duration, explosive activity.
- The more force a fiber generates, the less endurance it has.
- We cannot work more forceful fibers without also working less forceful fibers.
- The more forceful a fiber, the more metabolic benefit (fat-burning benefit) we get from exercising it.

## *Your Four Muscle Fiber Types*

Look at your biceps for a moment. The muscle you see is composed of tons of muscle fibers. Each human has four main muscle fiber types and each performs a unique role.

| | Produce little force/Greater endurance |
|---|---|
| Slow-twitch fibers | Type I |
| | Type IIA |
| Fast-twitch fibers | Type IIX |
| | Type IIB |
| | Produce more force/Lower endurance |

Type I muscle fibers allow us to do low-force work for a long period of time, like go for a 30-minute jog. At the opposite end of the spectrum, our type IIB muscle fibers allow us to do high-force work for a short period of time (say, jumping, lifting a heavy weight, or sprinting for 10 seconds). But here's the coolest part and just another reason why the All-Day Fat-Burning Diet's approach to exercise turns your body into a fitter, more athletic, fat-burning machine: When you perform a quick sprint or lift a heavy weight, you don't just work your type IIB fibers—you actually work the entire spectrum of muscle fibers!

Just as your body's energy requirements change when going from a slow jog to a sprint, a similar phenomenon occurs with your muscle fibers. For example, say you're about to do a set of pullups. Oh, dear! They're so tough, aren't they? But they're so good for you, too. As you attempt to pull yourself up toward the bar, your back, biceps, and shoulder muscles first try to generate enough force with their weakest type I fibers. When they don't generate enough force, the "cavalry"— your IIA fibers—is called in to help. However, let's say you're still struggling to pull yourself up. Now the stronger IIX fibers are brought in. They certainly help and get you closer to the bar, but you still need a little bit of a boost. And so your most powerful IIB fibers step in to help you over the top.

Thanks to the cumulative activation of all of your muscle fibers (known as orderly recruitment), heavier, challenging exercise actually enables you to work the most muscle possible. That's the secret to turning your body into a stronger, leaner, fat-burning machine. Oh, and it actually improves your health as well.

A study out of Boston revealed that doing exercise that recruited more type IIB fibers also improved insulin sensitivity and caused reductions in blood glucose, insulin, and leptin levels and that these effects occurred despite a reduction in physical activity.[31] Are you convinced yet that exercising in a way that recruits faster-twitch muscle fibers (such as short sprints and heavier lifts) is the ultimate way to burn fat and feed muscle? Remember, long, slow cardio (such as going for a 5K jog) requires little force and therefore works relatively little muscle. Of course, it's better than no exercise at all. The reality is that most exercise is good for you. But I'm obsessed with efficiency, and thus with which exercise is better, safer, and quicker at burning fat and making us stronger.

After all, I don't see much point to getting weaker, do you? But that's exactly what countless women are doing all over the world by spending most of their time doing aerobics classes and lifting 5-pound weights for 25 reps. This old-school mentality of "lift light to avoid bulking up" is complete nonsense. It wastes your time and makes you weaker. You might as well spend a week in outer space. If you're a woman who's been programmed to fear heavy lifting, then the following section will put that fear to rest for good. Lifting heavy works because it requires a lot of force and therefore works a lot of muscle, including our metabolically beneficial type IIB muscle fibers. Slowly lowering heavy weights (even your bodyweight) allows you to generate even more force, which increases your strength and requires less training volume.

The result is that you burn more fat, develop and maintain lean muscle, reduce your risk of injuries, and save a ton of time. What else could you do with your time if you only had to spend 90 minutes a week working out? Imagine having the strength and fitness level to play more in your daily life, whether that means outlasting your active kids or pursuing your own daily adventures. If you're a little older, just imagine the improvement in your quality of life as you're able to get off that comfy sofa more easily, climb stairs and carry groceries effortlessly, and get more stuff done around your house. The possibilities are endless, and it all starts with having a foundation of strength, not weakness.

## Ladies, Don't Worry: You Won't Bulk Up!

The vast majority of the hundreds of thousands of people I've helped over the past 2 decades were women: young, old, and in between. Not once have I seen an "after" picture where these ladies looked bulky or complained about getting too muscular from following my workout and nutrition recommendations.

Here's why: Everyone has a GDF-8 gene that controls a substance called myostatin, which in turn determines the amount of muscle we have. The base levels of myostatin and muscle in basically all women and most men make it impossible for them to naturally build bulky muscles. It does not matter how much resistance we use. The majority of us—especially women—do not have the genes to build bulky muscles via any form of exercise.

Additionally, women have only about 10 percent as much testosterone as men, and since it is the main muscle-building hormone, exercising for 90 minutes per week is certainly not going to turn you into a freakishly muscular bodybuilder.

Here are three workout options for you to choose from.

1. **Bodyweight Blast**
2. **Bodyweight Eccentrics**
3. **Eccentric Strength**

As you follow this program, I would strongly recommend that you cycle among these three workouts on your Regular-Calorie Days so that you tap into all their benefits and prevent your body from getting used to doing the same routine all the time. For pictures and video demonstrations of these workouts, plus some more advanced options, visit alldayfatburningdiet.com/resources.

### *Bodyweight Blast: Beginner*

## Protocol

1 set of each exercise for maximum reps (or hold where noted) within 1 minute

30 seconds of rest between exercises

1. **Pushups (from knees or feet)**
2. **Reverse Lunge Pumps**
3. **Plank**
4. **Reverse Pullups (requires Smith machine or other fixed bar)**
5. **Triceps Pushups (30 seconds of work per side)**
6. **Hamstring Pushoffs (requires bench or chair)**
7. **Side Planks (30 seconds of work per side)**
8. **Hip Thrusters (requires bench or stability ball)**

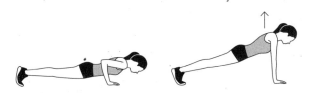

# PUSHUPS (FROM KNEES OR FEET)

**Muscles worked: chest, shoulders, triceps**

Place your hands on the floor so they're slightly outside shoulder-width. Spread your fingers slightly out and point them forward. Rise up onto your toes so that all of your body weight is on your hands and your feet, or your hands and your knees if that's too challenging.

Contract your abdominals to keep your torso in a straight line and prevent arching your back or pointing your bottom in the air. Bend your elbows and lower your chest down toward the floor. Once your torso is just above the floor, push up so that you return to starting position.

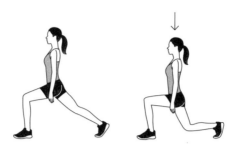

# REVERSE LUNGE PUMPS

**Muscles worked: legs**

To begin, stand tall with your hands at your side. Take a large and controlled step backward with your right foot. Lower your hips so that your left thigh (front leg) becomes parallel to the floor with your left knee positioned directly over your ankle. Your right knee should be bent at a 90-degree angle and pointing toward the floor with your right heel lifted.

Return to standing by pressing your left heel into the floor and bringing your right leg forward to complete one rep. Alternate legs, and step back with left leg. Continue alternating for required reps.

 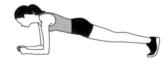

# PLANK

**Muscles worked: core**

Get into a pushup position on the floor, then bend your elbows 90 degrees and rest your weight on your forearms. Your elbows should be directly beneath your shoulders, and your body should form a straight line from your head to your feet. Tighten and draw your abdominal muscles in (as if putting on a tight pair of pants), squeeze your glutes and legs, and hold for required time.

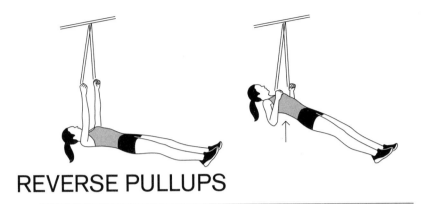

# REVERSE PULLUPS

**Muscles worked: back, biceps, forearms**

Lie on the floor underneath the bar (which should be set just above where you can reach from the ground). Grab the bar with an overhand grip (palms facing away from you). Contract your abs, and try to keep your body in a completely straight line.

Pull yourself up to the bar until your chest touches the bar. Lower yourself back down and repeat.

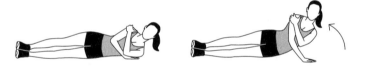

# TRICEPS PUSHUPS

**Muscles worked: triceps**

Lie on your left side with your body in a straight line and the palm of your right hand planted on the floor just under your left shoulder. Put your left arm across your chest and grab your opposite shoulder. Use your left triceps muscles to push your entire upper body off the floor so that only your legs and hips remain on the floor. Return to the start. Finish the set with that arm and then switch sides.

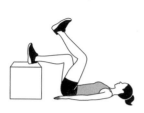
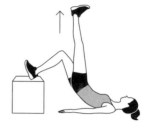

# HAMSTRING PUSHOFFS

**Muscles worked: hamstrings, glutes**

Lie on the floor with the heel of your right foot on a chair or bench (make sure it's stable or up against a wall). Come into a bridge position, lifting your pelvis off the floor and driving your left leg in a straight line toward the sky. Lower back to floor and repeat for required reps, then switch legs.

# SIDE PLANKS

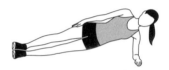

**Muscles worked: core**

Lie on your left side with your legs straight. With your left forearm directly under your left shoulder and abdominals contracted, prop yourself up so that all of your bodyweight is supported by your left forearm and your body forms a diagonal line. Rest your right hand on your hip. Hold for required time, then switch sides.

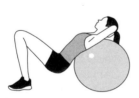
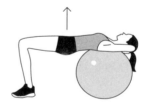

# HIP THRUSTERS

**Muscles worked: glutes**

Sit on the ground with your back against a stability ball, feet planted firmly in front of you and hip-width apart. Squeeze your glutes together and raise your hips off the floor so that your body forms a straight line from your shoulders to your knees (parallel to floor), and then slowly descend back to the ground. Repeat for required reps.

## *Bodyweight Eccentrics: Beginner*

### Protocol

4 reps for each exercise

Tempo = 1—0—6 (1-second push or pull, no pause, 6 seconds to return to start)

30 seconds of rest between exercises

2 sets

1 minute of rest between sets

1. **Pushups (from knees or feet)**
2. **Reverse One-Leg Drop Squats (requires box or bench)**
3. **Side Plank Drops**
4. **Dead Bug (with or without stability ball)**
5. **Split Lunges**
6. **Supine Alternating Leg Lowers (2 on each side)**

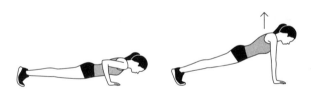

# PUSHUPS (FROM KNEES OR FEET)

**Muscles worked: chest, shoulders, triceps**

Place your hands on the floor so they're slightly outside shoulder-width. Spread your fingers slightly out and point them forward. Rise up onto your toes so that all of your bodyweight is on your hands and your feet, or your hands and your knees if that's too challenging.

Contract your abdominals to keep your torso in a straight line and prevent arching your back or pointing your bottom in the air. Bend your elbows and lower your chest down toward the floor. Once your torso is just above the floor, push up so that you return to starting position.

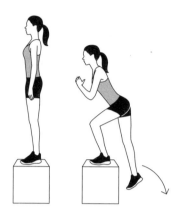

# REVERSE ONE-LEG DROP SQUATS

**Muscles worked: legs**

Stand on a box or stable bench, then sit back and lower your right leg off the back of the box/bench toward the floor so that you end up in a single-leg squat position on your left leg. Just before the right leg touches the floor, use your left leg to push yourself back up to a standing position. Repeat for required reps then switch legs.

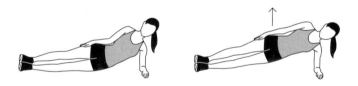

# SIDE PLANK DROPS

**Muscles worked: core**

Lie on your left side with your legs straight and your right hand resting on your hip. With your left forearm directly under your left shoulder and abdominals contracted, prop yourself up so that all of your bodyweight is supported by your left forearm and your body forms a diagonal line. Slowly lower your left hip to the floor and lift back up to top position. Repeat for required reps.

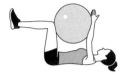
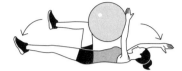

# DEAD BUG

**Muscles worked: core**

Lie flat on the floor on your back while holding a stability ball. Contract your abdominals and raise your legs off the floor at a 90-degree angle so your lower legs are parallel to the floor. Raise your arms straight to the sky so they're parallel to your thighs. Simultaneously lower your left leg and right arm until they are just off the floor and pause for a second before returning to start position. Repeat for the leg and arm on the other side. This is one repetition.

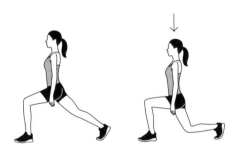

# SPLIT LUNGES

**Muscles worked: legs**

Stand tall and then step your left foot out approximately 3 feet in front of your body. Your stance should be long enough so that the heel of your back foot is off the floor. Slowly bend your left knee, lowering your body toward the ground. Your left knee should be bent at a 90-degree angle, with your foot directly under your knee, and your right knee should be just above the floor at its lowest point. Now, use the muscles in your legs to push yourself back up to your standing split stance (hence, you're not coming back up to a full feet side-by-side standing position). Repeat for required reps, then switch legs.

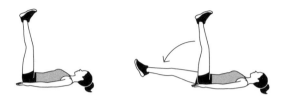

# SUPINE ALTERNATING LEG LOWERS

**Muscles worked: core**

Lie flat on your back with your arms at your sides and both legs straight up in the air over your hips. Keeping your left leg straight, slowly lower your right leg down to the floor. Return to the starting position and repeat with your other leg. Continue alternating for the prescribed number of repetitions.

## *Eccentric Strength: Beginner*
## Protocol

4 reps for each exercise @ 85 to 90 percent max weight

Tempo = 1—0—6 (30 seconds to finish each set)

1 minute of rest between exercises and sets; 2 minutes of rest between supersets (1a/1b, 2a/2b, 3a/3b)

2 sets

**1a. Sumo Squats**

**1b. Dumbbell or Bench Presses**

**2a. Romanian Deadlifts (with dumbbells or bar)**

**2b. Alternating Reverse Shoulder Presses**

**3a. Chinups (or Lat Pulldowns)**

**3b. Ab Wheel (or Ball) Rollouts**

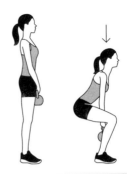

# SUMO SQUATS

**Muscles worked: legs**

Use a squat rack for this exercise. If you do not have a squat rack, use a kettlebell or dumbbell between your legs, as illustrated. To begin, first set the bar on a rack that best matches your height. Once the correct height is chosen and the bar is loaded, step under the bar and place the back of your shoulders (slightly below the neck) across it.

Hold on to the bar using both arms at each side and lift it off the rack by first pushing with your legs and at the same time straightening your torso. Step away from the rack and position your legs using a wider-than-shoulder-width stance with your toes slightly pointed out. Keep your head up at all times (looking down will get you off balance), and also maintain a straight back.

Slowly lower your body by bending your knees (as if sitting back into a chair) as you maintain a straight posture with your head up. Continue down until your thighs are parallel to the floor. Return to standing by pushing the floor with the heels of your feet as you straighten your legs again and go back to the starting position. Repeat for the recommended number of repetitions.

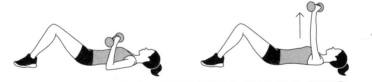

# DUMBBELL OR BENCH PRESSES

**Muscles worked: chest, shoulders, triceps**

To perform dumbbell chest presses, refer to the instructions on page 141.

To perform bench presses, lie back on a flat bench with the bar overtop the middle of your chest (just below your collarbone). Place your hands on the bar so that your elbows form a 90-degree angle. Lift the bar from the rack and hold it straight over you with your arms locked. Slowly lower the weight until the bar just about touches your middle chest.

Push the bar back to the starting position as you breathe out. Focus on pushing the bar using your chest muscles. Lock your arms and squeeze your chest in the contracted position at the top of the motion, hold for a second, and then start coming down slowly again. Repeat the movement for the prescribed amount of repetitions.

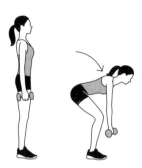

# ROMANIAN DEADLIFTS (WITH DUMBBELLS OR BAR)

**Muscles worked: glutes, hamstrings**

Put a barbell (or two dumbbells) in front of you on the ground and grab it using a pronated (palms facing down) grip with your hands a little wider than shoulder-width apart. Bend your knees slightly and keep your core strong and back straight. Keeping your back and arms completely straight at all times, use the back of your legs/hips to "pull" the weight off the ground and up to the front of your thighs so that you're in a standing position. Once you are standing completely straight up, keep your core strong and lower the weight back to the floor by pushing your hips back, only slightly bending your knees. Repeat for the recommended amount of repetitions.

# ALTERNATING REVERSE SHOULDER PRESSES

**Muscles worked: shoulders, triceps**

Stand with your feet shoulder-width apart and core and glutes contracted. Hold a dumbbell at each shoulder. Now, press both weights above your

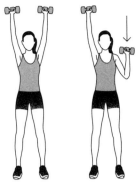

shoulders, keep the right arm straight (holding the weight), and lower the left arm/weight to your left shoulder. Press the left arm/weight back to top, hold, and lower the right arm/weight. That's one repetition. Repeat for required number of reps.

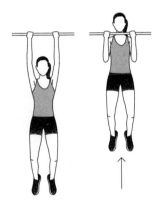

# CHINUPS (OR LAT PULLDOWNS)

**Muscles worked: biceps, back**

To perform lat pulldowns, refer to the instructions on page 142.

To perform chinups, grab the pullup bar with your palms facing your torso and your hands closer than shoulder-width apart. Pull your torso up until your head is around the level of the pullup bar. Concentrate on using your biceps muscles in order to perform the movement. Keep your elbows close to your body. After a second of squeezing your biceps in the contracted position (at the top), slowly lower your torso back to the starting position so your arms are fully extended. Repeat this motion for the prescribed amount of repetitions.

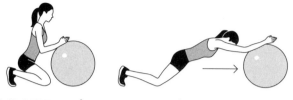

# AB WHEEL (OR BALL) ROLLOUTS

**Muscles worked: core**

Kneel on the floor and hold the Ab Roller with both hands (or place your forearms on a stability ball) in front of you. Slowly roll the ab roller (or ball) straight forward, stretching your body out as far as you can go. Be sure to contract your core muscles and eliminate any curvature in your lower back to focus the effort on your core muscles. After a pause at the stretched position, start pulling yourself back to the starting position as you breathe out. Repeat for the required number of repetitions.

## DAY 5: LOW CAL

### *Rest or Active Recovery*

Your Low-Calorie Day is another opportunity to give your body a break and allow it to recover. After all, the combination of the interval speed burst and full-body metabolic conditioning workouts plus your bodyweight and eccentric strength workouts is more than enough intensity to take on three times a week. Burnout and overtraining occur when you fail to understand the importance of rest and recovery. That's not to say that you should sit around doing nothing in between workouts. You should certainly be lightly active, walking and doing micromovements throughout the day. (We'll explore these micromovements in the next chapter.)

The point here is that if you're exercising effectively, with sufficient loads, your body will be begging for time off and you won't want to do much more than move slowly for a couple of days afterward. Honor your body by giving it the tender love and care that it requires to repair and bounce back stronger.

## CHAPTER 7

# STEP 5: REST YOUR WAY TO FASTER FAT LOSS

One day before I wrote this section, I was at the gym getting ready to go through a terrific strength workout—one of my favorites, in fact: deadlifts and kettlebell presses. That's it. Just those two exercises done for numerous sets with heavy weights, very few reps, and a focus on good tempo for strength development. I did a comprehensive warmup before I started and loosened up my muscles using a foam roller. After a few warmup sets, I added more weight to the bar for my deadlifts, ready to tear into my first set. I felt good, and I distinctly remember visualizing myself performing each rep with ease and perfect form. Then, it happened.

On my third set, as I was lifting 205 pounds—a weight that I could normally deadlift four or five times—I felt a pop. I immediately dropped the weight to the floor and found a way to stand up straight. I couldn't believe it yesterday, and I can't believe it now: I tweaked my lower-back muscles—the erector spinae. I'm going to have to take it easy for the next few weeks, modifying any workouts I do to accommodate this injury.

This little accident is serving as inspiration for what I'm about to write. It's very easy to find books and articles on different workout regimens, but far fewer tell you what to do in between workouts. Recovery is just as important as the workouts themselves, as it can prevent these kinds of injuries from happening. Based on this most recent experience, I want to devote a few more pages than I'd originally planned to this very topic.

Getting injured is never fun, but it's even more annoying when you've just started a new workout plan. Imagine if you got a week and a half into this program and strained your hamstring; not only would you not be able to work out, but there's also a chance you might put on a little more weight than you started with, thus defeating the very purpose of buying this book. We don't want that to happen! So it's very important that you learn some clever ways to help your body recover, including gentle ways to keep it moving.

## WHY YOU NEED A RECOVERY ROUTINE

As I've shared with you, you won't be exercising every day on this program. It's simply not productive and may, in fact, be harmful. However, that doesn't mean you'll be completely sedentary on your days in between workouts. If you want to avoid the kind of injury I just experienced, and even minimize soreness between workouts, it's important that you move every day.

I'll never forget learning about something called creep in my third-year university sports medicine class. According to this concept, solid materials have a tendency to move slowly or deform permanently under the influence of mechanical stresses. In plain English this means that most structures can bend and deform under a certain load after a certain amount of time. And depending on the magnitude of the applied stress and its duration, the deformation may become so large that a component can no longer perform its function.

Try holding a spoon off the edge of a table and placing a 1-pound weight in the spoon. The spoon will quickly bend and deform. If you instead add a lighter load, the spoon might not deform immediately, but given enough time it may end up bent and useless as well. Creep also applies to the human body. Sitting at a desk all day, hunched over your computer, is the same as putting weight in the spoon and hanging it off of the table—eventually, your body will deform. Maybe it already has. Take a look around your office, or even the supermarket next time you're there—I'm sure you'll notice many people without very good posture.

This is why daily movement is so important. Sitting or even standing in the same position for prolonged periods imposes a load on your muscles and other tissues that, over time, can shift them from their default setting. If you spend most of your time sitting with your legs bent at 90 degrees, then both your hip flexors and hamstrings are spending most of their time in a shortened state. It's no wonder, then, that flexibility becomes a major issue for so many people.

When you work out, you create trauma within your muscles. This stimulus helps them grow and get stronger. Very often, because the muscles are contracted so heavily in a workout, they can feel stiff for a few days afterward. A number of physiological processes are going on here, but to keep things simple, the more contracted your muscles, the shorter and stiffer they will become. What happens when you flex your biceps? The muscle goes from a lengthened state to a shortened, or concentric, one. If your muscles are constantly shortened due to over-training or prolonged sitting, for example, then they are less likely to regain their natural length.

For instance, too much chest training or prolonged periods of hunched sitting with your shoulders rounded forward will shorten your pectoralis major and minor (chest) muscles. Since one of them (the pec minor) attaches to your collarbone, if it shortens, it will then pull your entire shoulder girdle down and forward. The result is the rounded, hunched shoulders commonly seen in seasoned office workers as well as many male gym rats who obsess about getting a "bigger chest" without doing an appropriate amount of upper back work to counteract the forward pull of the pec minor muscle. So how does this relate to fat loss?

This example illustrates what happens to your body if you sit around all day and expect a few short workouts per week to make up for it. There are 168 hours in a week. If you work out for maybe 3 or 4 of them, what are you doing with the rest of that time? Let's say you spend 60 hours sleeping; that leaves you with 104 waking hours. Maybe 30 or 40 of those hours you're sitting at your work desk or on the couch, leaving 60 to 70 hours. What should you do with that time to promote fat loss and counteract the effects of all that sitting?

## THE IMPORTANCE OF MICROMOVEMENTS

Exercising less with the right intensity is key to losing fat, but so, too, is simply moving your body more on a regular basis. Walk. Take the stairs. Do a few pushups here and there. Do 10 bodyweight squats before you eat. Pick up your kids. Run to the mailbox. Do some lunge walks down the hall. Get up out of your chair every 15 minutes and stretch. All of these micromovements add up over time and can help you burn more calories and avoid turning into the hunchback of Notre Dame. After all, the human body does not become weak and decrepit because of the aging process; it gets that way because we become lazy and fail to provide adequate stimulation for it to continue getting stronger and working at its best.

For instance, it's been well established that daily exercise such as walking for 30 minutes yields substantial health benefits and that regular physical activity attenuates the health risks associated with overweight and obesity.[1] In fact, a large 20-year study in Sweden found that, among 7,142 men, those who were most physically active during leisure time had a lower risk of death from heart disease, cancer, and all causes.[2]

Another way to consider the importance of regular movement is by understanding a simple equation from physics.

### Work = Force x Distance

This is the single most important tool I use when talking about how your body can burn more calories and thus fat. Here, work represents how many calories your body burns. Force is the amount of weight moved, and distance is, well, the distance covered.

Based on this equation, you end up doing more work if you either:

- Move more weight (that's why we lift heavier in our workouts) or
- Move a given weight over a greater distance (that's why we use full-body movements)

It's really that simple. Knowing this, you can see why a 400-pound person will likely lose more weight than a 150-pound person following the same exercise plan. The former simply has much more weight (force) to carry over the same distance. Let's compare three simple scenarios of basic physical activity. Again, these are completely separate from your focused, intense workouts.

**Scenario #1:** You weigh 200 pounds and spend all day sitting.

**Scenario #2:** You weigh 200 pounds and walk 10,000 steps (5 miles, or 8,000 meters) per day.

**Scenario #3:** You weigh 200 pounds and walk 10,000 steps per day wearing a 10-pound knapsack.

Intuitively, you probably know which scenario will yield the most work and thus burn the most calories, right? Scenario #3, because the amount of force generated is greater over the same distance as Scenario #2. In order to help you move more consistently, I've included a little challenge below for you to follow.

## The Micromovement Challenge

- Do 25 bodyweight squats first thing in the morning when you get up.
- Plank for the duration of one commercial break when you're watching TV.
- Run to the mailbox or to the nearest stop sign.
- Run up and down the stairs three times each day.
- Do 10 pushups before breakfast, lunch, and dinner.
- Stand up and do 5 lunges after every 20 minutes of sitting.

Will you take me up on the challenge?

Most people gain weight over several years or decades because of small, unconscious habits (eating one or two chocolates a day, grabbing a Starbucks milkshake—er, I mean Frappuccino—every morning, etc.). You can reverse that trend and lose that weight by incorporating some of these micromovements into your day. Keep in mind that these movements are not a replacement for your workouts. They are simply tools to keep your body active throughout the day.

As a baseline during this program, you should be walking at least 30 minutes every day. However, walking should not be considered your workout; it's basic physical activity. When it comes down to it, it's a foundational requirement just like breathing is for bringing oxygen into your body. There should be no negotiation. No matter what, find a way to walk every single day. Get a dog if you have to.

But there's even more you can do.

## MOBILITY EXERCISES AND DEEP-TISSUE WORK

Have you spent a few minutes before a workout or sporting event stretching because you thought you were loosening up your muscles? I'm sure you've seen professional athletes doing the same. Sad to say, it's an archaic method of preparation and really doesn't do much good at all. What does work, however, are mobility exercises and deep-tissue work, as they improve your range of motion and work out built-up tension throughout your body, respectively. You can think of them as being a part of the same "movement family" as your daily micromovements. Better yet, think of these two strategies as having a personal physiotherapist and massage therapist on call 24/7.

It boggles my mind when I see elite athletes and seasoned gym goers stretching for 20 minutes before their workouts. It's not that stretching is terrible, but it's been well proven at this point that if you're going to stretch, you should do it when your body is warm, not before your workouts. Instead, this is the time to be getting your body mobile, loose, and limber. Other than doing static stretching during your yoga class or on its own when your body is warm, stretching is pretty much dead. It really doesn't help much with mobility, and worse yet, it can significantly hinder your workout performance and even increase your risk of injury.

A 2013 study in the *Journal of Strength and Conditioning Research* examined two groups performing either a dynamic warmup or static stretching before a maximal lift workout. The study found that the latter suffered a significant decrease in strength and stability during the subsequent workout.[3] In another recent (and massive) study, researchers pooled data from 104 studies on this topic and conclusively found that static stretching before activity should be avoided because it decreases strength and power.[4]

So why do we continue to stretch before physical exertion? I guess it's because we feel it's going to prevent an injury, but that's really just another myth that needs to be busted. A review in the *Clinical Journal of Sport Medicine* of a number of other studies revealed that there is no injury-preventing benefit to doing any form of static stretching before a workout. And in the studies that do show any benefit, it's usually because a proper warmup was done as well.[5]

Why does stretching hamper performance and not make you bulletproof to injury, even though we've been told otherwise for decades? Well, we don't fully understand, but part of the problem is that stretching actually does loosen muscles and their accompanying tendons. However, in the process, it also makes them less able to store energy and spring into action. Plus, having lax muscles and joints is not what you want before activity. You want stability and support.

When you're doing *dynamic stretching*, you're not just lengthening a specific muscle like you do with static stretching. Instead, dynamic stretching incorporates exercises that take you through ranges of motion to improve posture control, stability, and balance and get your muscles warm for the upcoming workout. If you want to feel more supple, then mobility work is imperative, especially when you've spent a lot of time sitting on your butt, which, if you think about it, is actually a form of static stretching. Hold one position for any length of time and certain muscles will stretch while their opposing muscle groups will shorten.

The good news about dynamic stretching is that it doesn't have to be done only when you work out. Heck, I start every single morning with some form of dynamic-stretching routine. Here are a few of my favorites.

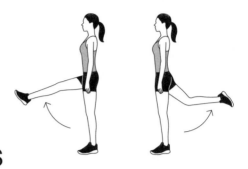

# LEG SWINGS

**This is a great movement for opening up your hips and hamstrings.**

Hold on to a wall or fixed surface (or do this move without support for an added stability challenge). Swing one leg back and forth as if you're kicking a soccer ball. Do about 10 swings on each side.

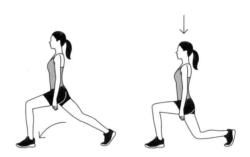

# LUNGE WALKS

**Since this movement exaggerates the walking, running, or walking up stairs motion, it has a lot of everyday applications and increases mobility throughout your entire hip area.**

Step forward using a long stride, keeping the front knee over or just behind your toes. Lower your body so that your back knee hovers just above the floor. Then push forward, take a giant step, and repeat with the opposite leg.

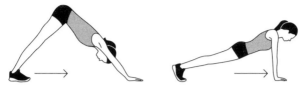

# INCHWORMS

**These might actually be my favorite dynamic exercise of all time, as they target the entire backside of your body and open up a lot of muscles that get stiff with prolonged sitting. It's actually a dynamic version of vinyasa flow yoga.**

> Starting in a Downward Dog position on your hands and feet, walk your feet as far forward as possible while keeping your legs straight. Then, walk your hands out, extending your body into a pushup position, and lower toward the floor, arching your back so that your head and shoulders reach to the sky. Then, flow back into Downward Dog. Walk your feet in again and repeat 5 times.

So what does any of this have to do with burning fat? Everything. After all, taking care of your body is essential for feeling good and being in optimal condition on a day-to-day basis. It creates a scenario in which you feel like working out on a consistent basis. See, when I tweaked my low-back muscles after that deadlift workout I mentioned earlier, I was sidelined for about a week. All I did was ice, heat the area (with a hot water bottle), do daily mobility exercises, foam roll, massage the muscles, and anything else that could speed the recovery process and help me stay limber.

But I certainly couldn't work out. And if you're sidelined due to injury or just feeling sore all the time, then you certainly won't want to work out either. That becomes a problem because it tips the scale in favor of you storing more calories, instead of burning them. You have to take care of your body.

Considering all that I've said about stretching and even the Downward Dog pose, you might be wondering: Is yoga worthwhile or a waste of time?

You might be surprised, but I'm actually a huge fan of yoga, especially hot yoga. I've done yoga for more than a decade now, and although I don't spend 3 hours a day going to yoga class like I used to, I still do my own version on most days. And really, just a few minutes is all you need. But again, do this separately from your workouts. I prefer to do my yoga routine first thing in the morning. It limbers up my body, focuses my mind, and helps me kick off the day just right. Actually, you'll never guess where I've made the most use of yoga: It was during my time working with the men's soccer team at the University of Toronto.

I'll never forget the first session I took the team through. In front of me, I had 22 guys who were as stiff as boards and looking at me like my name was Charles Manson. We gathered in a big circle around the middle of the field, me in the center, leading the way. At first, many of the guys tried to smother their laughs as I took them through Downward Dog and various flows. Then, after we finished our 20-minute session, they were shocked at how good they felt. Their legs felt lighter, many aches and pains had diminished, and their minds were more focused.

I sold our coaching staff on the need to do yoga with our team three times per week. We started preseason, and by the time our season had begun, not a single one of our starting players was sidelined. It was a much different picture than in the past, when nearly half our team, at some point of the season, was sidelined with a preventable injury. By doing regular yoga just three times per week, we reduced injury rates by 82 percent! Combined with a smart conditioning program I had the guys follow during the off-season, we were stronger and more resilient than ever. It just so happened that we won the provincial (state) championship that year and finished fourth at nationals. Not bad, if you ask me.

Yoga is terrific, and it can actually be a form of dynamic stretching if you move through the poses in a fluid manner. So by all means, enjoy it to the fullest. Plus, the stress-relieving powers of yoga cannot be overlooked. Anything that lowers stress in your body will help turn it into a fat burner instead of a fat storer.

# USING COLD THERAPY FOR RECOVERY

As a former pro athlete and strength and conditioning coach for top athletes, I can tell you firsthand that ice is necessary for speeding up recovery from injury since it reduces unwanted, prolonged swelling and inflammation. Not only that, but it can also be very beneficial for recovering from intense exercise. That said, this has been a controversial area over the last few years, and the science is split—some studies show no benefit of cryotherapy on recovery while others do show a benefit.

Here's my experience: When I was the strength and conditioning coach for men's soccer at the University of Toronto, one of the most important recovery strategies that kept our players healthier, less prone to injury, and "lighter" feeling was implementing optional ice baths after training and games. We had a very compact 3-month season, which involved training 5 days per week with two games on the weekends. Recovery was obviously paramount. Although it was a bit of a shock to their systems at first, most of the players fell in love with jumping in the ice bath for a few minutes after a hard session.

If you're reading this, you're probably not a pro athlete, and I sure don't think you need to take an ice bath after your workouts. However, it's still good to know that cold can help your body recover so that you don't feel stiff and sore all the time. Even something as simple as taking a cold shower or lowering the temperature in your house can help. And if you're not a fan of cold showers, then you can always take a hot-cold ("contrast") shower, where you alternate between hot and cold water, which gets the blood flowing in and out of your muscles to speed removal of exercise-induced waste products, like lactic acid.

A 2008 study in the *European Journal of Applied Physiology* looked at the effect of cold water immersion, hot water immersion, and contrast water therapy on delayed onset muscle soreness (DOMS). Thirty-eight men completed two experimental trials separated by 8 months. One trial involved an intense exercise bout (to cause muscle damage), followed by passive recovery and one of the three hydrotherapy protocols for 72 hours after exercise. These protocols were done for 14 minutes postexercise.

The results showed that both cold water immersion and contrast water therapy were effective in reducing the physiological and functional deficits associated with DOMS, with both fostering improved recovery of isometric force and dynamic power (measured by improved jump squat performance) and reducing localized swelling.[6] I don't know about you, but I'll take any unfair advantage I can to help my body recover from intense exercise. And if it also helps me burn more fat and better my health, then that's even better.

## EASING YOUR MUSCLES WITH DEEP-TISSUE WORK

Although it's important to keep your muscles in motion, that motion doesn't always have to be strenuous. In fact, you don't even have to be the one putting your muscles through their paces. In between workouts, I recommend various forms of deep-tissue work that alleviate muscular tension and make you feel great. Massage, active release technique, and Rolfing are just a few examples.

By all means, make use of them if you can, although I don't expect that everyone has the money to pay a massage therapist on a regular basis. Thankfully, you can do some of the very same work before and after your workouts with a cheap foam roller. Yes, it's really that easy. For less than $30 you can buy a cylindrical piece of hard foam that will do the trick. I have one, and I consider it to be my personal massage therapist. If you don't have a foam roller, you can still get started today by using a simple tennis ball to roll out your points of tension. There really is no reason to complain about being stiff and sore all the time when you have simple options like this.

When your body has chronic tightness, tension, or an area with a history of injury or overuse, adhesions usually form in the muscles, tendons, and ligaments. These adhesions can block circulation and cause pain, inflammation, and limited mobility. This is known as the cumulative injury cycle (or cumulative trauma disorder). It means that a repetitive effort such as sitting or lifting a weight causes certain muscles to tighten. But here's the dilemma: A tight muscle tends to weaken, and a weak muscle tends to tighten. This creates a vicious cycle.

As a result of weak and tight tissues, internal forces arise. Friction, pressure, or tension can be present at the same time, which then reduces bloodflow to the area. With less circulation, less oxygen comes to the tissue, causing fibrosis and adhesions to occur in the affected tissues. Eventually, a tear or injury occurs, and this restarts the adhesion process. That's why lifting the groceries out of the car didn't tweak your back. It was likely the years of sitting that created weak and tense tissues that were just waiting to snap.

Stretching does nothing to alleviate this. However, deep-tissue work does. It is simply the act of physically breaking down these adhesions, usually by applying direct deep pressure or friction to the muscles. As these adhesions are broken down by deep-tissue work, bloodflow and lymph flow to the affected area are enhanced. Instead of driving to a massage therapist several times per week, you can whip out your foam roller in the comfort of your own living room and work through your body's tight spots while watching your favorite TV show. My foam roller is an integral part of our family. It has its own place in the corner of our living room. It's almost ornamental. That way, it's accessible and I see it regularly, which reminds me to use it every day.

There are many types of foam rollers on the market, but I recommend getting one that is very firm. Avoid the cheap ones that are nothing more than glorified flotation noodles like you find in many swimming pools. You can also get a little more adventurous and use a RumbleRoller, which is essentially a foam roller with protruding extensions that dig deep into your muscles. They're certainly quite uncomfortable—but highly effective.

When it comes to your workouts, here's the sequence I recommend.

1.  **Light aerobic warmup**
2.  **Foam rolling**
3.  **Dynamic stretching**
4.  **Workout**
5.  **Cooldown with more foam rolling**

Breaking up tension in your muscles is a good idea before you start hammering them again with heavy weights. In fact, a 2014 study

## Sue's Story

"I needed to lose a lot of weight because, among other reasons, my excess weight was causing back and knee problems. But at the age of 74, losing weight is not an easy thing to do. I have tried many different eating plans but always just lost a few pounds, then seemed to gain it back overnight, and often more with it.

"I was thrilled that I got to try this program with the prospect of possibly doubling my weight loss. I don't eat a lot and generally eat healthy; however, I had never tried a program such as this one where I cycle how much I eat each day.

"In just 21 days, I lost 12 pounds. I reduced my waist and hips each by 4.5 inches. I am very happy so far with this program and am grateful to Yuri for creating it. I also slept better during the program, did not really have any cravings, and found the food choices to be really good. Thank you, Yuri!"

showed that foam rolling before a workout improved hip and hamstring range of motion.[7] Once you combine it with some dynamic-stretching exercises, you'll feel like a million bucks. You'll be able to dive into your workout knowing that you're less prone to injury.

After your workout is another opportunity to relieve built-up tension. This is not the time to stretch. After all, tension in your muscles is much like a knot in a rubber band—the more you stretch it, the tighter the knot gets. Again, save the stretching for another time. After a workout is when you should take a few minutes to cool down and bring your body back to a more relaxed state. You want to bring those stress hormones down. Follow your 5- to 10-minute cooldown with another few minutes on the foam roller, and you'll feel amazing.

A 2015 study in the *Journal of Athletic Training* looked to see if foam rolling after a workout could alleviate muscle fatigue and delayed onset muscle soreness and improve physical performance. Participants performed two workouts 4 weeks apart, involving 10 sets of 10 squats at 60 percent of their 1-repetition maximum (that's a lot of volume). They followed that up with either no foam rolling or 20 minutes of foam rolling either immediately or 24 hours or 48 hours postexercise. The researchers found that foam rolling improved quadriceps muscle tenderness by a moderate to large amount in the days after training. Sprint times also improved, as did strength-endurance, following the foam rolling.[8]

As effective as foam rolling and deep-tissue work are, I should warn you that deep-tissue massage (whether hands-on or via a foam roller) is not a comfortable, relaxing experience. The pressure and friction that deep-tissue work involves can be pretty intense. The best way to get through it is to breathe deeply and remind yourself that you're doing your body a big favor. The tension will dissipate with just a few sessions, and with time you'll feel so much better afterward. You should also be prepared for the possibility of soreness after deep-tissue work, because as the pressure breaks up adhesions and introduces friction into an affected area, your tissues will probably get the same type of inflammation-related fluid accumulation you get when you lift weights.

But now you also know that one of the best ways to alleviate the soreness is by using cold therapy. Take a cold shower or dunk your legs in cold water for a few minutes. You can even take an Epsom salt bath if you want something warmer and more relaxing. The salts in the bath are essentially magnesium sulfate, which can penetrate the skin and relax a lot of built-up tension.

———

What I hope you've gathered from this chapter is this: Relaxation is paramount when you're on a regular exercise routine. However, because the human body was designed to move, it's important for us to stay in motion, even when we're recovering. The more you move, the less stiff you will be, and considering that the ultimate stiffness is rigor mortis, that's something you want to avoid as much as possible! Staying in motion, quite literally, is what gives us life.

CHAPTER **8**

# STEP 6: SLEEP YOUR WAY THIN

W hat's the one thing everyone wants more of but can never seem to get enough of? If "money" was your answer, you're not wrong, but that's not the answer I'm looking for. Given the breakneck pace of modern life, I'd argue that sleep is the hot commodity so many of us are desperate for.

Day in and day out, we shuffle through endless errands like zombies, daydreaming about *actually* dreaming in the comfort of our beds, far removed from the world and its worries. I know it sounds like I'm exaggerating, but the Centers for Disease Control and Prevention agrees with me. In 2012, the organization reported that nearly a third of Americans were sleep deprived, and in 2014 it declared that insufficient sleep was a public health epidemic![1] So, be honest with yourself: When was the last time you had a full, restful night of sleep?

As much as everyone loves to sleep, we too often skimp on it. After all, when you have a million and one things to do, it's very easy to underestimate the importance of the one time of day when you can't do anything at all. That's a huge mistake, because even though you may not be ticking off items on your to-do list while you're snoozing, your body is actually performing a number of critical functions, including:

- Regenerating, growing, and repairing itself
- Consolidating new learning
- Cleaning up cellular garbage

We spend roughly one-third of our lives asleep, so sleep must be important, right?

What's more, sleep is essential to our mission in this book: helping you to lose weight. Here's a wake-up call: A good night's sleep goes a long way toward helping you stay trim, and without it, all your exercise and healthy eating may be nearly useless. For that reason, it's imperative that you understand the dynamics of sleep and the role it plays in weight maintenance.

# SLEEP 101

The science of sleep is fascinating because it illustrates how connected we are to the natural world. For all our modern technology, from cell phones to drones, we are still animals programmed to rise with the sun and sleep when it sets. Like many animals on the planet, we evolved to get most of our sleep at night because that's when it's generally colder. Were we awake and active from sundown to sunrise, our bodies would have to expend more energy to keep warm.

Our bodies have become wired this way thanks to a tiny region in the brain very close to our optic nerves called the *suprachiasmatic nucleus (SCN)*. It controls our circadian rhythm, which you've probably heard of before. The circadian rhythm is your internal clock, which flows in accordance with the rising and setting of the sun, dictating when you feel alert or sleepy. This internal clock is so important that it gets better blood supply than any other part of the brain and is nearly impossible to destroy, even in the event of a stroke.

The SCN's placement right by our optic nerves is very significant, as light plays a crucial role in steering our circadian rhythm. When it's light outside, the suprachiasmatic nucleus sends a signal to your pineal gland to raise your cortisol levels and drop your level of melatonin, the sleep hormone. At night, this is reversed: Cortisol drops and melatonin rises, preparing us for a night of sleep. Simultaneously, our body temperature lowers in sync with the temperature outside. As you can see, we are biologically hardwired into a deep relationship with nature.

Except when we're not. The constantly running motor of modern life is much different than what our ancestors experienced 200,000-plus years ago, and with it have come numerous forces that interfere with the way we sync our own internal rhythms with nature. Let's explore just how you are unsuspectingly disrupting the quality of your sleep.

## HOW LIGHT AFFECTS YOUR SLEEP PATTERN

What's the last thing you did before you went to sleep last night? Can you remember? Odds are you toyed with your phone, watched television, or spent some time staring at a screen. We devote so much of our daily life to screens these days, whether we're checking our e-mail or texting our loved ones. Unfortunately, if you're doing this right before bed, you're also disrupting your natural sleep cycle.

The blue light emitted by the various screens you use so regularly has the same effect as daylight on your circadian rhythm. They both qualify as *zeitgebers*, environmental or external cues that regulate your biological cycles. The alarm clock that screams at you every morning? That's a zeitgeber. The screeching cats outside your window or even the timing of your meals every day? They're zeitgebers as well. If you're fiddling with an app on your phone or watching a television show right up until you hit the hay, its blue light has sent a message to your brain that you're not ready to sleep. This can make getting to sleep difficult and prevent you from getting a good night of sleep. I'm sure this sounds odd to you, but the effects of blue light are not to be underestimated.

A 2014 study performed at Brigham and Women's Hospital gathered 12 subjects and instructed six of them to read on an iPad for 4 hours before they went to sleep for 5 nights in a row. The remaining six subjects were instructed to read printed books by dim light for the same period of time. The groups switched tasks after a week. The results were quite clear: The researchers observed that those reading on an iPad took longer to fall asleep and also released lower levels of the sleep hormone melatonin. Their melatonin release was delayed by 1 hour, and they reported feeling groggier and sleepier than their book-reading counterparts the next morning. The results remained the same when laptops, cell phones, and some e-readers were used in place of the iPads. Who knew texting or checking Facebook could be so harmful?[2]

It's not just the light from your electronic devices that you have to be mindful of, however. Your access to daylight plays a significant role in the consistency of your sleep patterns, as well as your mood and energy. This is light you want to be exposed to as much as possible. It's perhaps the main reason I enjoy walking with my dogs first thing every morning: It gives me the energy I need for the day ahead and prepares me for a more restful sleep when bedtime rolls around.

A perfect example of light's impact on your sleep cycle is jet lag. For instance, when I travel from Toronto (Eastern time) to Los Angeles (Pacific time), I gain 3 hours. A 5-hour flight leaving Toronto at 9:00 a.m. means I arrive in Los Angeles at 11:00 a.m. local time (or 2:00 p.m. Eastern time). This is great because I get an extra 3 hours in my day! However, by dinnertime my body is ready for bed. Remember, I normally go to bed around 10:00 p.m., which means 7:00 p.m. in Los Angeles. The next morning is even trickier. If I normally wake up at 5:00 a.m. back home, I could be waking up at 2:00 a.m. in LA.

I'm sure you've experienced this time zone conundrum. The first few days can really be uncomfortable. But the cool part is that you can actually speed your adjustment—or readjust your internal circadian clock—by immediately immersing yourself in the local environment. Experienced travelers are quite familiar with this hack: If you arrive in the morning, get outside and take in all that natural sunlight, even if it's bedtime back home. If you arrive at night, then do your best to wind things down and get ready for bed. Within a few days, your body will have adapted to your new time zone.

I'm sure this will have you thinking differently about your light intake, but it's not the only thing that affects the quality of your sleep.

## HOW QUANTITY AFFECTS QUALITY OF SLEEP

It's often said that we should aim for 8 hours of sleep a night. It's not a strict rule, but it's a good target. People's need for sleep varies slightly and lessens as we age. For instance, newborns require the most sleep (12 to 18 hours) because they're growing and learning at an exponential rate, while most adults require about 7 to 9 hours, based on the latest research from the National Sleep Foundation.[3]

There's a sweet spot when it comes to sleep. A University of California, San Diego, study of more than one million adults found that people who live the longest report sleeping for 6 to 7 hours each night.[4] Another study of sleep duration and mortality risk in women showed similar results.[5] As with exercise, too much of a good thing can definitely be a bad thing. A 2005 study in the journal *Hypertension* found that sleeping more than 7 to 8 hours per night has been consistently associated with increased mortality.[6] On the opposite end of the spectrum, getting too little sleep creates a "sleep debt" that must be repaid in the following days; otherwise, you end up living your life in a state of mental and physical fatigue.

Since sleep is a time for repair and recovery, you would think more sleep would be required if your body were hurting or inflamed. At least, that's my theory, especially considering that when I cleaned up my diet and my body and started taking care of myself, my requirement for sleep greatly diminished. Now, I sleep about 7 hours a night and feel great all day long—no naps required.

Optimal *amount* of sleep is perhaps not as meaningful as the *timing* of that sleep in relation to our circadian rhythm. The research seems to indicate that for adequate and fully restorative sleep to occur, the following two circadian markers must occur after the middle of the sleep episode and before awakening: maximum concentration of the hormone melatonin and minimum core body temperature.[7] And, as we've learned, this mainly happens at night. Nighttime is also when we're best able to

## LIGHT, SLEEP, AND BODY TEMPERATURE

A 1992 study by the American Physiology Association quickly shifted the sleep schedules of male subjects by 12 hours to accommodate eight or more consecutive simulated night shifts.

In the study, the men were exposed to artificial light of approximately 5,000 lux (a unit of brightness) for 3 to 6 hours each night, slept at home in very dark bedrooms during the day, and wore dark welder's goggles whenever they went outside during daylight—a 180-degree shift from what their bodies were used to.

Their body temperature was continuously measured, and daily questionnaires provided estimates of sleep time and mood.

What's fascinating about the results of this study is that the men's circadian temperature rhythm shifted by approximately 2 hours per day, for a total of a 12- to 16-hour shift by the end of the study. Earlier, I mentioned how low body temperature was a prerequisite for the onset of good sleep. Normally, that happens at night. But this study showed that by looking at artificially bright light at night (when it's normally supposed to be dark), these men shifted their body temperature from its normal tendency to be low at night to being low at other times of the day.[8]

reach the most prized sleep state of all: deep sleep.

Human growth hormone is released during deep sleep, and interruption of this stage abruptly stops its release. As we've seen throughout this book, HGH is one of your best friends when it comes to staying lean because it promotes fat loss and improved muscle growth and repair. Deep sleep, intense exercise, and fasting all raise growth hormone in the body. Now you know why all three are important components of the All-Day Fat-Burning Diet.

The shift in and out of deep sleep happens at certain times of the night regardless of when you go to bed. So if you hit the sack very late (like after midnight), your sleep will tilt toward lighter, non-deep sleep (known as REM sleep). And that reduction in deep, restorative sleep may leave you groggy and blunt-minded the next day. Over time, it can also impair your body's ability to repair and recover, especially if you're exercising regularly.

In my college years and when I was playing soccer competitively, I never thought about sleep at all. I wouldn't mind partying with friends until dawn or sleeping in until noon. I had no regular schedule. Had I known this information back then, I'm sure it would have made a big difference in my performance and how I felt on a day-to-day basis. Now that I'm in my midthirties and much wiser, I've realized that sleep is critical for my day-to-day productivity and overall functioning. Plus, with three young boys, the only way I can get stuff done is when they're out of the house or asleep. In fact, most of the writing of this book occurred between 5:00 and 7:00 a.m. I'm a big believer that the early morning is when our best creativity surfaces, so I've built my life around waking up early. It's a priority for me. Thus, I go to bed between 9:30 and 10:00 p.m. and wake up at 5:00 a.m.—every single day. That's up to 7.5 hours of sleep.

I would recommend getting to bed before 11:00 p.m. for the best-quality sleep, which means you should naturally wake up earlier as well. And keep in mind that if you've taken a nap during the day—especially a longer one that may have tapped into deep sleep—your drive to sleep will be lessened. So work with your body to see what fits. Not every human being is best suited to going to sleep by 10:00 p.m.

## WHY SLEEP CONSISTENCY MATTERS

Of all the obstacles to good sleep you've learned about in this chapter, this might be the most damaging: not establishing an early and consistent bedtime. It sounds funny, doesn't it? Bedtime is for kids, right? We adults have so many things to do, and we can't retire for the night until they're all done, correct? The answer to that is a firm, undebatable *no*. Sleep consistency is one of the most powerful things you can do to establish and maintain a healthy circadian rhythm.

A 2011 study in the journal *Sleep Medicine* examined the effects of an advanced sleep-wake schedule in 25 adults with typical late-sleep schedules who also had subclinical symptoms of delayed sleep phase disorder (DSPD). That's a condition in which sufferers have disrupted circadian rhythms, generally fall asleep hours after midnight, and have difficulty waking up in the morning. Here, participants were kept on individualized, fixed, advanced 7.5-hour sleep schedules for 6 days. They were exposed to either blue light (group 1) or dim light (group 2) for an hour upon waking each day. The results? After just 6 days, both groups showed significant circadian phase advances, meaning that these 25 adults were now falling asleep earlier and waking more naturally.[9] And this was after just 6 days of staying on a fixed sleep schedule!

As for early bedtime, a study from Rush University Medical Center may shed some light (no pun intended) on this question. This study compared the effect of 7 to 19 nights with a late bedtime (1:00 a.m.) versus 7 to 19 nights with an early bedtime (10:00 p.m.) on the body's melatonin rhythm. Remember, melatonin helps us fall asleep. Each of the subjects was woken (lights on) at 7:00 a.m., then exposed to at least 5 minutes of outdoor light between 7:00 and 8:00 a.m. each day. The researchers found that despite the morning light exposure, the release of melatonin following the late bedtime nights was delayed by almost 45 minutes compared with the early bedtime nights. This suggests that when we truncate our sleep by going to bed later (past 10:00 p.m.), we significantly impair our body's natural rhythm and melatonin response, which negatively affects our sleep.[10]

You may think that everything you have to take care of is more important than getting to bed early, but that's just not true. If anything, by maintaining a consistent, relatively early bedtime, you'll sleep better and be more productive every day. I assure you of that.

## HOW SLEEP SLIMS YOU

By this point, it should be clear that poor sleep isn't good for you, but that's not why you bought this book. Let's address what you're really concerned about: how all this affects your weight-loss efforts.

Remember, back in Chapter 1, we looked at how insufficient or poor-quality sleep is strongly related to weight gain? At a very basic level, sleep deprivation is a big-time stressor on your body. And we've seen that chronic stress eventually scares your body into holding on to weight. This all goes back to our primal origins, when chronic stress meant starvation or death. Thus, the body is built to hold on to fat as a protective mechanism just in case we run out of food. Yes, I know— this makes absolutely no sense in our modern world, but remember, we're still using the same operating system that was given to our earliest ancestors.

A fascinating study out of Canada (called the Quebec Family Study) revealed that both short and long sleeping times predict an increased risk of future weight and fat gain in adults. This 6-year study involved 276 adults ages 21 to 64 and looked at changes in adiposity (fat storage) among short-sleeper (5 to 6 hours), average-sleeper (7 to 8 hours), and long-sleeper (9 to 10 hours) groups. After adjustment for age, sex, and baseline body mass index, short-duration sleepers gained 1.98 kilograms (4.3 pounds) more and long-duration sleepers gained 1.58 kilograms (3.5 pounds) more than average-duration sleepers did over 6 years. Short- and long-duration sleepers were also 35 percent and 25 percent more likely, respectively, to experience a 5-kilogram weight gain compared with average-duration sleepers over the 6 years. And the risk of developing obesity was elevated 27 percent for short- and 21 percent for long-duration sleepers compared with average-duration sleepers![11]

A 2010 review of the literature in the journal *Obesity Reviews* scoured 79 studies on this topic and found that the ". . . studies showed that short sleep duration is consistently associated with development of obesity in children and young adults."[12] These findings are illuminating. You might think that packing on a few pounds in 6 years as a result of too little or too much sleep is no big deal, but when you compound that weight gain with the other lifestyle factors mentioned throughout this book, you can start piecing together this weight-gain puzzle that you and millions of others are trying to solve.

So what are we going to do about it? We're going to start sleeping much better. That's all there is to it. Here, I'm going to unleash some powerful sleep wisdom on you that you should apply, starting tonight. Deal?

## Set Consistent Sleep and Wake Times

You know the deal here: Figure out what time you need to wake up each morning. And then, based on the 7 to 9 hours of sleep required for good health and a lean body, determine what time to go to bed each night. Your goal should be to maintain this schedule every day of the week, so find a way to make this work for you. I'm telling you, it's the single most powerful way to reset your circadian rhythm and reestablish healthy hormone levels in your body—both of which directly impact your ability to lose weight.

## Turn Down the Lights

To recap: Melatonin is a naturally occurring hormone controlled by light exposure that helps regulate your sleep-wake cycle. Because its production is controlled by light exposure, your brain should secrete more in the evening when it's dark, to make you sleepy, and less during the day when it's light and you want to stay awake and alert. Melatonin is what makes you feel sleepy and ready for bed, so you want to minimize anything that disrupts its natural secretion cycle. That includes:

- Spending long days in an office away from natural light
- Basking in too many bright lights at night, especially from your TV, computer, or mobile device screens

Ideally, you want to eliminate any source of unnatural light at night. Thus, at least an hour before bed, I challenge you to turn off your TV, shut down your computer, and power off your smartphone. I know it sounds difficult, but give it a try. Spend more time in the darkness before going to bed. If you want to read, then do so with a reading lamp that uses a red-light bulb, since red-light wavelength does not disrupt our melatonin and sleep cycle like blue light does.

In fact, check this out: In a 2006 study, researchers looked at brain activity during sleep in eight young men after 2 hours of evening exposure to light. The findings revealed that after blue-light exposure, the amount of deep sleep was reduced in the first stage and increased during the latter stages of the sleep cycle. This is the opposite of what should normally happen during high-quality sleep. Moreover, blue light significantly shortened rapid eye movement (REM) sleep duration during the various sleep cycles.[13]

If you need to be on your computer at night (okay, okay, I admit I do it myself sometimes), then at least install a free app called f.lux (get it at justgetflux.com), which dims your computer screen and reduces its blue-light emission. Alternatively, you can use a pair of BluBlocker sunglasses around the house at night. Yes, you'll look like a maniac, but it'll allow you to get your TV, cell phone, and computer fix without compromising the quality of your sleep. (Just don't let anyone see you.)

## Create a Relaxing Bedtime Routine

Given how hard you work, you deserve to be pampered. It serves a real purpose, too: If you make a consistent effort to relax and unwind before bed, you will sleep easier and more deeply. A peaceful bedtime routine sends a powerful signal to your brain that it's time to wind down and let go of the day's stresses. We often create a bedtime routine with our kids but fail to do so for ourselves. If reading our kids a bedtime story and recounting moments of gratitude can work for them, it can surely work for us, too.

Here are a few relaxing bedtime rituals to try.

- Read an inspiring book by a soft light (red light is best).
- Take an Epsom salt bath.
- Meditate and/or visualize.
- Engage in gratitude journaling.
- Listen to soft music or guided meditation/visualization.
- Do some easy stretches or foam rolling.
- Listen to books on tape.
- Script your upcoming day.

I personally use a combination of these techniques every night (other than the bath, which is rare for me), and here's why: First, by writing down what you're grateful for, you train your mind to focus on what is great in your life instead of what is negative. That's way more uplifting than watching the news before going to bed, which is a terrible idea if having a positive outlook on life is important to you. Along with giving and contributing, feeling grateful is one of the only sustainable ways to feel happy and fulfilled in life. And when you feel this way, you're more likely to engage in activities that are in line with your higher self and your major goals. When you feel crappy and focus on what's wrong with your life, you end up making decisions that make you feel good in the moment, like eating a bag of greasy, fattening chips.

Second, by meditating and visualizing what you want your life to be like, you program your subconscious mind to find ways to make that a reality in the physical world. Never forget the power of your mind. Everything in the external world started in someone's internal world. This book was once a mere idea of mine; now it's in your hands. You wouldn't have a car if Henry Ford hadn't dreamt up the mass-market automobile. Every single material object on this planet started as an esoteric idea in someone's mind. You have that same ability to create whatever you want—whether that's a strong, lean body or the business of your dreams.

I know this may sound "airy-fairy" and "woo woo," but you're missing the boat if you're not mentally scripting your life. I don't know a single high-level athlete who does not use visualization. Athletes do it because the brain does not know the difference between something it vividly imagines and something it actually experiences. That's why meditation is one of the most powerful practices you can add to your daily life. There really is no right or wrong way to meditate. Were you to just sit on your couch and breathe deeply for a few minutes each day, you'd start experiencing some of its amazing benefits. Countless studies have shown the health and de-stressing benefits of meditation, and considering how chronic stress forces the body to hold on to weight, I'm sure you can understand why I'm recommending it.

Meditation has also been shown to provide many of the same benefits as sleep. On top of that, it's also been shown to improve the quality of our sleep, especially when done prior to bedtime. Here are just a few ways that it helps your brain, your body, and the quality of your sleep.

- Studies of long-term transcendental meditation (TM) practitioners have shown that TM slowed breathing and decreased heart rate, both responses of deepened relaxation.[14]

- Slow-wave sleep (deep sleep) and REM sleep have both been shown to be enhanced in those who practice meditation. An increased number of sleep cycles (indicating better-quality sleep) has been observed, along with the fact that older meditators can restore deep-sleep states that normally lessen with age while retaining the sleep pattern of younger nonmeditating people.[15]

- Meditation calms the nervous system, allowing for parasympathetic predominance (which creates relaxation) among both experienced meditators and novice meditators with less practice.[16]

- Meditation has also been shown to regulate the hypothalamic-pituitary-adrenal (HPA) axis and thereby the release of the stress hormones cortisol and epinephrine, while increasing favorable hormones like growth hormone, thyroid-stimulating hormone, melatonin, and serotonin.[17, 18, 19]

Need more proof that regular meditation is good for you? I didn't think so.

Research tells us that insomniacs are distinguished from those who sleep easily by high levels of anxiety and physiological arousal. If this sounds like you, in addition to the mental relaxation techniques described above, you may want to incorporate muscle relaxation before bedtime. A study of 18 insomniacs found that just six half-hour muscle relaxation training sessions helped them fall asleep 23 minutes faster than those who did no muscle relaxation before bed.[20] And the cool part is that muscle relaxation can be built into your meditation or visualization practice. Here's a simple way to do it.

- Lie in bed and get comfortable.
- Forcefully contract your muscles and hold that contraction for a few seconds.
- Then, relax your muscles.
- Repeat.

The contrast of the contraction and relaxation brings greater awareness of what your body should feel like when it's relaxed and what it feels like when it is tense and stressed. Give it a shot tonight.

## Make Your Bedroom Sleep-Friendly

Light, temperature, noise, and sleeping surface. These are the external variables you want to control to the best of your ability. A cold "tomb" is what you want for the best sleep. Based on what you now know about melatonin, hopefully you realize that complete darkness is the name of the game for good sleep.

Here are a few tips to help you darken your room.

- Cover electrical displays (such as alarm clocks and phone lights).
- Use heavy curtains or shades to block light from windows.
- Try a sleep mask to cover your eyes.
- Use a flashlight to go to the bathroom at night. That will keep the light to a minimum so it will be easier to go back to sleep.

You want your room to be relatively cool. Typically, a temperature between 60°F and 67°F makes for the best sleep. Your bedroom should also be free of any noise. This is easier said than done, especially if you have a baby or live on a busy street. If that's the case, try using earplugs that can block out the noise.

Make sure your mattress is comfortable and supportive. The one you have been using for years may have exceeded its life expectancy—about 9 or 10 years for most good-quality mattresses. Have comfortable pillows and make the room attractive and inviting for sleep, but also free of allergens and objects that might cause you to slip or fall if you have to get up during the night. Whether you want a hard or soft mattress and pillows is up to you so long as your choice is conducive to better, deeper sleep.

## Wake Up to Natural Light (or Simulated Natural Light)

You've been sleeping deeply for 7 hours when, all of a sudden, you hear a loud, annoying beeping. It sounds like it's drilling itself into your brain! You leap up to smash the off switch on your alarm clock and sit on the side of the bed, feeling like you've just been clobbered in the face with a frying pan. Is that a relaxing way to wake up, or is your body's fight-or-flight stress response firing on all cylinders? I think you know the answer.

I'm not a fan of these scare-you-out-of-bed alarm clocks. I hide them in the closet whenever I'm in a hotel room. Naturally, the best solution is to wake up with the rising sun, but if you're sleeping in a very dark room, you won't know when the sun is up. The other option you have, and the one I've used for quite some time now, is a sunlight-simulating alarm clock. These alarm clocks emit a light that gets progressively brighter over 15 to 20 minutes, reaching their brightest by the time you want to get out of bed. Many also feature nature sounds like chirping birds or ocean waves to make you feel like you're sleeping outside. It's such a better way to wake up in the morning, as you can imagine. No matter what time you set your alarm for, you feel so much more at peace as you get out of bed to start your day. I personally use the Philips Wake-Up Light. It has single-handedly transformed my mornings and made waking early so much easier.

Once you're up, be sure to get outside. Few things will wake you up as well as the warm, bright sun. Unfortunately, that's not an option if it's wintertime, but there's a solution for that. When I realized that my body didn't cope well in the long, dark days of winter—especially

## DON'T UNDERESTIMATE THAT MORNING LIGHT

Light, or the absence of it, can have a big effect on your mood as well. A study in the journal *Science* looked at the effect of bright light exposure in eight patients who regularly became depressed in the winter (as day length shortens).

Mood and markers of depression significantly improved after just 1 week of exposure to bright light in the morning. This antidepressant response to morning light was accompanied by earlier nighttime melatonin production, which is so important for good sleep.[21]

when I wake up at 5:00 a.m.—I started using bright light therapy every morning upon waking. For me, this involves using a 10,000-lux bright light for 2 to 3 hours each morning. As of this writing, I've been using NatureBright's SunTouch Plus light for 18 months, and I can tell you that it makes a huge difference. I feel more awake in the morning, since bright light supports the natural morning surge in cortisol. And by nightfall, my body is much better prepared to sleep.

Here are a few more ways to reestablish your body's natural circadian rhythm.

- Remove your sunglasses in the morning and let light into your eyes.

- Spend more time outside during daylight. Try to take your work breaks outside in sunlight, exercise outside, or walk your dog during the day instead of at night.

- Let as much light into your home or workspace as possible. Keep curtains and blinds open during the day, and try to move your desk closer to the window.

## NUTRITIONAL CONSIDERATIONS FOR ENHANCING YOUR SLEEP

A number of neurotransmitters in the brain are involved in the sleep-wake cycle. Therefore, it is possible that what you eat—especially later in the day—can act upon these neurotransmitters and influence your quality of sleep. Remember, everything in your body ultimately comes from the foods you eat. Your skin, hair, eyes, and everything inside your body, including your hormones and neurotransmitters, owe their existence to the raw materials you put into your body—the food you eat.

Diet obviously influences your central nervous system, partly through the production of serotonin and melatonin. Synthesis of serotonin is dependent on the availability of its precursor in the brain, the amino acid L-tryptophan (Trp).[22] Tryptophan is transported across the blood-brain barrier by a system that shares other transporters, including a number of large neutral amino acids (LNAAs). Thus, the ratio of Trp/LNAAs in the blood is crucial to the transport of tryptophan into the brain. You can increase this ratio by taking pure tryptophan or tryptophan-rich protein (spirulina, game meat, eggs, spinach, halibut). By the way, turkey contains no more tryptophan than other kinds of poultry; in fact, turkey actually has slightly less tryptophan than chicken. So, feeling tired after eating Thanksgiving dinner is likely the result of the massive onslaught of food that wears on your digestive vitality, rather than the turkey itself.

The ingestion of other forms of protein generally decreases the uptake of tryptophan into the brain, as it becomes the least abundant amino acid and, therefore, other LNAAs are preferentially transported into the brain. However, as I mentioned earlier, carbohydrates actually increase tryptophan in the brain by driving more amino acids into your muscles through the stimulation of insulin (which stores energy). With more amino acids in the muscle and less in the blood, the result is an increase in free tryptophan, which can then cross the blood-brain barrier.[23] Once in the brain, tryptophan becomes the precursor to the relaxing neurotransmitter serotonin, which then gets converted into melatonin.

Only a small number of studies have investigated the effects of meals or drinks of varying composition on sleep. One study examined the effects of high-energy versus low-energy liquid lunches (993.5 versus 306 calories), compared with no meal, on daytime naps. Both liquid meals caused subjects to experience increased time in stages 2 and 3 of non-REM sleep when compared with no meal. However, there were no differences in how quickly subjects fell asleep.[24]

Again, there is very limited research in this area, though it appears that reduced caloric intake may result in poor sleep. Interestingly, in my experience and that of many of my clients, quality of sleep tends to improve after a day of fasting. This is only anecdotal, so you'll have to see for yourself whether having little to no food or a lot of food makes a difference in your sleep.

Overall, the research seems to indicate the following associations between food and sleep.

- Foods with a high glycemic index (GI), such as white rice and potatoes, may promote sleep. However, they should be consumed more than 1 hour prior to bedtime and, ideally, closer to 4 hours earlier. This is yet another reason I recommend increasing your carb intake as the day progresses. Yes, it seems counter to what others have told you in the past, but this tends to work best for your body.

- Diets high in carbohydrate may result in shorter sleep latencies (the time it takes to fall asleep).
- Diets high in protein may result in improved sleep quality.
- Diets high in fat may negatively influence total sleep time.
- When total caloric intake is decreased, sleep quality *may* be disturbed.
- The hormone melatonin and foods that have a high melatonin concentration may decrease sleep onset time.

You should now have a better sense of what and when to eat at night: some protein and fat, with perhaps more carbs, with dinnertime ideally 4 hours before bedtime. Additionally, ensuring that your overall diet is generally higher in protein can help the overall quality of your sleep. The best part is that you don't need to obsess about this stuff because my 5-Day Food-Cycling Formula and the 21-day meal plan that I've laid out for you in this book have done the work for you.

## DOES EXERCISE IMPROVE YOUR SLEEP?

By now, you might be wondering how exercise impacts your sleep. So let's take a quick look at how and when to work out to create the best possible sleep results.

As you probably know, high-intensity exercise revs up your body and leads to a surge of stress hormones like adrenaline (epinephrine) and cortisol, so doing this type of exercise close to bedtime might not be the smartest idea. A meta-analysis conducted by the American Psychological Association looked at 38 studies of the effects of exercise on sleep. Results showed that exercise's impact on sleep latency, slow-wave sleep, REM sleep, and total sleep was moderate. The more significant finding was that intense exercise closer to bedtime impaired the ability to fall asleep.[25]

A more recent study looked more closely at time of day of exercise and its impact on sleep. Here, subjects were asked to perform maximal aerobic exercise (the "beep test"—basically, progressively faster running) at both 2:00 p.m. and 8:00 p.m. The findings revealed that sleep-onset-latency, number of awakenings, slow-wave sleep, and REM sleep latency were all negatively affected after the evening test session.[26] This is not surprising, and I'm sure you can relate if you've ever engaged in evening sports or like to work out after work. One of the reasons I no longer play competitive amateur-level soccer is that most of the games are either at 7:00 p.m. or 9:00 p.m. For years, playing at these times would ruin my next day. I'd get home by midnight and not be able to sleep for hours. The next day was a complete write-off.

Now, I value my sleep and consistent sleep-wake schedule much more than playing soccer until all hours of the night. But that's just me. If playing on a sports team or working out at night is your only option, then that's certainly better than doing nothing at all. The most powerful recommendation I can make is to do a good cooldown, followed immediately by meditation or some other form of relaxation. Doing so will lower the stress hormones circulating in your body that impair sleep and lower your core temperature—both of which will help you turn in for a good night's sleep.

Okay, that's a pretty comprehensive look at sleep. By now, you should have a solid understanding of the health and fat-loss implications of poor-quality sleep, how to set up your house and lifestyle to get better sleep, and specific nutrition and exercise recommendations to get deeper Zs. I really can't stress this enough: Sleep is the most important component of your recovery. No matter how active you are during the day, a good night's sleep is essential to functioning as you should while you're awake. Commit yourself to it alongside the other tasks in this book, and I guarantee you'll gradually start waking up slimmer in no time at all.

We've just walked through 6 steps to a slimmer, happier you. As straightforward as this outline is, however, I know that you'll need further support to get where you want to be.

So many aspects of getting and staying in shape are often overlooked, be they social or emotional. There are also matters of habit and convenience. I've accounted for all of this, and in the next section,

## Deborah's Story

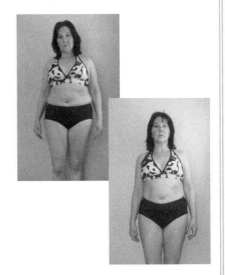

"By following this program, I lost more than 11 pounds and 10 inches in 6 weeks. I'd say that's a success! When I first went into nursing school 20 years ago, I gained 20 pounds. I think I gained 10 more with every degree I got thereafter. I've tried many, many diets over the years: the cabbage soup diet, low carb, low cal, yeast free, detox diets—you name it! My weight loss had been minimal, and I always gained the weight back because it was not something I could sustain over time. What I've learned from this experience is that I can still lose weight by following this plan with some breaks here and there. I see this as something I can continue long term. Thank you, Yuri!"

we'll lay out a series of tips, hacks, and support structures that will carry you through to the body you want to see in the mirror.

I'll also condense everything we've already mapped out into a quick reference guide that you can refer to throughout your 21 days. Forgot today's workout plan or eating schedule? It's all in there.

Best of all, I'll share with you the smoothies and meals that will delight your palate over the next 21 days, and hopefully will become a part of your regular diet in the weeks and months to come. They're all regulars in my household, and they make eating healthy, fun, and yes, even comforting.

Are you ready? This is where it all comes together.

 Part III

# How to
# Eat Your
# Way Thin

## CHAPTER 9

# START YOUR FAT-BURNING ENGINES

Here we are: the heart of this program. So far in these pages, we've worked through the damaging things happening to your body every day because of the litany of unhealthy living and eating habits you've likely practiced for years. In the next 21 days, we're going to rip these habits all apart and start again. This 3-week plan combines the diet, exercise, and recovery protocols introduced in earlier chapters. It's one I've tested and fine-tuned over years of working with clients. I can confidently say that when implemented correctly and consistently, it will supercharge your metabolism, optimize your health, and help you lose weight on autopilot.

Obviously, each person's results will vary, but you can look forward to losing up to 5 pounds per week. Best of all, you won't experience the usual sense of deprivation and confusion that a new diet or exercise program brings on. As complicated as the world is, staying healthy and lean is rather simple. I'll prove it to you. Actually, you'll prove it to yourself. Ready? Let's do this!

# STEP 1: DETERMINE YOUR BASELINE

The basis of this plan is a 5-day cycle of eating and exercise that you'll repeat over the next 3 weeks (and beyond, if you can). It's made up of five different days: a Low-Carb Day, a 1-Day Feast, a 1-Day Fast, a Regular-Calorie Day, and a Low-Calorie Day. Since we've already covered each day in detail, here, I'll provide an abbreviated look at how to eat on each day.

You've probably heard a number of definitive "truths" about how much you should eat at any given meal, all backed up by "experts." Some tell you to count calories. Others say you should weigh your food. Pretty meticulous, no? If you ask me, it's really a bother, and I know you don't need those complications. The easier alternative I offer to you is the Serving Size Simplifier, first mentioned in Chapter 5. You're not going to put your food on a scale or calculate how many calories it contains. Instead, you're simply going to eyeball it.

If this seems lax, don't worry. It's actually a remarkably easy and effective way to ensure you're getting the right amount of food every time you sit down to eat. If you're following the recipes in this program, the portion sizes will already be taken care of for you, for the most part. These guidelines will become increasingly handy (no pun intended) when preparing your own meals from scratch and also when eating in restaurants.

## *The Serving Size Simplifier*

### *Thumb = Fit Fats*

For fat-dense foods like oils, butters, nut butters, nuts, and seeds, use your entire thumb to determine your serving size. I recommend 1 to 2 thumb-size portions of fats with most meals for women and men, respectively. So your total intake, by day, will look like this:

Low-Carb Day = 4 thumb-size portions (women)/8 thumb-size portions (men)

1-Day Feast = 5 thumb-size portions (women)/10 thumb-size portions (men)

1-Day Fast = none

Regular-Cal Day = 3 thumb-size portions (women)/6 thumb-size portions (men)

Low-Cal Day = 3 thumb-size portions (women)/6 thumb-size portions (men)

## Palm = Protein

Low-Carb Day = 3 palm-size portions (women)/4 palm-size portions (men)

1-Day Feast = 2 palm-size portions (women)/3 palm-size portions (men)

1-Day Fast = none

Regular-Cal Day = 2 palm-size portions (women)/3 palm-size portions (men)

Low-Cal Day = 1 palm-size portion (women)/2 palm-size portions (men)

## Fist = Starchy Carbs and Fruit

Low-Carb Day = up to ½ fist-size portion

1-Day Feast = at least 3 fist-size portions (women)/4 fist-size portions (men)

1-Day Fast = none

Regular-Cal Day = 2 fist-size portions (women)/3 fist-size portions (men)

Low-Cal Day = 1 fist-size portion (women)/2 fist-size portions (men)

## Hand Bowl = Fibrous Veggies

Here's a little secret: There's actually no maximum serving size for fibrous veggies—salads, green leafy vegetables, or cruciferous vegetables. They're loaded with amazing nutrients and very few net carbs and calories, meaning you can eat as much of them as you want.

That said, there is a minimum. Fibrous veggies are such a crucial part of this plan that you don't have the option of skipping them except during your 1-Day Fast. For maximum effect, load up on veggies, and try to eat quite a bit more than the bare minimums listed below. (For easy reference, a hand bowl is the bowl formed when you cup both hands together; 2 hand bowls equals the size of a small bowl of salad.)

**Minimums**

Low-Carb Day = 2 hand bowls

1-Day Feast = 3 hand bowls

1-Day Fast = none

Regular-Cal Day = 2 hand bowls

Low-Cal Day = 2 hand bowls

You might not have noticed, but there's actually a formula at work here: The amount of food you eat on your Regular-Calorie Day is your baseline. The amount you eat on your feast day is 50 percent more than you'd ordinarily eat, and the amount you eat on your Low-Calorie Day is 25 percent less. You'll be amazed at how well this simple system works.

## Lyn's Story

In just one round of the All-Day Fat-Burning Diet—3 weeks—Lyn lost a whopping 12 pounds! Here's what she had to say.

"I like the variety. I love several of the menu items including the morning smoothies, which are a mainstay for me, and I also love the chili and the tomato soup. I like knowing the day's food, so I can even make plans with friends, knowing ahead what type of food I can eat, which is better than just trying to fit something in. Most other eating plans are boring, but the variety made it fun, and if I wasn't eating carbs one day, I knew I could have them in a couple days. I feel better and can think much more clearly, and I just don't have the emotional highs and lows I used to. I just feel good overall."

# STEP 2: EAT AT THE RIGHT TIMES

Just as you've received a great deal of confusing inherited wisdom regarding how *much* you should eat, there's a great deal of junk floating around out there about exactly how *often* you should eat. Some experts say you should eat no fewer than five or six times per day—otherwise your metabolism will "shut down." Others say that eating far less is necessary for weight loss. Those are the two extremes, but there are plenty of other eating timetables in between. At this point, I wouldn't be surprised if there are some diets that tell you to eat only when there's a full moon!

The truth is that you should eat only when your body tells you to. As I've found time and time again, the truth about anything is often very simple, and the same goes for eating. I have only two rules for you to follow.

1. **Eat when you're hungry.**
2. **Stop when you're 80 percent full.**

That's it.

For years, we've been led to believe that there was some magical meal frequency that would speed up our metabolisms, control our insulin and cortisol levels, and manage our appetites. However, a recent review of the literature in the *Journal of the International Society of Sports Nutrition* suggests otherwise.[1] In a nutshell, all that matters is that you eat the right foods in the right amounts. Once you're doing that, meal frequency is really just a matter of personal preference. You can eat lots of small meals each day, eating every few hours, or eat a few big meals each day with bigger time gaps between them. It's not rocket science. Eat when you're hungry. Stop when you're 80 percent full.

Your body always tells you what it needs at any given time, but we've become so disconnected from ourselves that we don't understand the signals it sends us. By listening to your body, you'll know how much or how little to eat. Similarly, you'll also know if you're legitimately hungry or feeling tempted to eat out of anxiety or depression.

As a general rule of thumb, your biggest meal of the day should come right after you work out (except on your Low-Carb Days). That's when your muscles are hungriest and most receptive to nutrients. After you've put them through their paces, you also need to replenish the carbohydrates they store. Aside from that, meal timing has very little impact on your ability to burn fat.

Here's a confession: Most mornings, I don't even eat breakfast. Sure, I know it's considered by many to be the most important meal of the day, but that simply doesn't work for me. I'll regularly go for several hours on water with apple cider vinegar or even a green juice, and come lunch, I'll have a big smoothie, salad, or leftovers from the previous day. Evenings are generally when I load up with a big dinner. That's what works for me. It may not work for you, but only you can determine that.

You have to think of yourself as both scientist and subject, conducting a series of experiments on yourself, making notes along the way. You're not looking to transform yourself into Frankenstein's monster, but rather a lean, optimized version of your current self. The results you get along the way should be your guide. For example, if you're eating five or six times a day and still not looking and feeling the way you want, it's time to try something different.

Maybe you need to start your day with a big workout, followed by a substantial breakfast and fewer calories throughout the rest of the day. Perhaps you skip breakfast entirely, have a small lunch, and dig into a hearty dinner. It really doesn't matter. You simply have to determine what works best for you. I know that might be hard to get your head around after a lifetime of eating three square meals a day or more recent indoctrination into some newfangled eating regimen. For that very reason, I've laid out a 21-day meal plan with an array of recipe and meal-timing options. You can follow them to the letter or not. All you have to do is follow the food guidelines for that day; however, how you choose to break that food up into meals and snacks is entirely up to you.

Actually, there's one more thing you have to keep in mind, and it's quite important: At night, it's best to finish your last meal at least 2 to 3 hours before hitting the sack. Far too many of us like to enjoy a little (or not-so-little) snack before bed, but it's not a healthy habit if you're trying to lose weight. As harmless as it may seem, that quick snack alters the balance of your hunger hormones, leptin and ghrelin, which affect melatonin, insulin, and thyroid function.

Confused? Let me map it out for you. Here's what normally happens at night:

1.  **You eat dinner and, a few hours later, your blood sugar and insulin levels fall.**

2.  **Decreasing insulin triggers the hormone leptin to be released to inhibit hunger when you go to bed.**

3.  **Leptin triggers thyroid hormone release to keep you warm and burn stored fat during the night. This process is balanced with melatonin release, which induces sleep.**

Now, if you eat close to bedtime, this normal process gets thrown out of whack.

1.  **You'll have trouble sleeping.**

2.  **The next day, your lack of sleep decreases insulin sensitivity and causes a prediabetic situation in which you have much lower glucose tolerance.**

3.  **Insulin will be elevated, and you will be less sensitive to leptin.**

4.  **You will be hungrier because the hormone ghrelin will be elevated. You'll particularly crave foods higher in sugar due to your poor blood sugar state.**

5.  **You'll have less desire to be active, leading you to burn fewer calories on the days after short sleep.**

I bet you didn't think a few cookies or a little leftover spaghetti before you hit the hay could have such an impact on your body chemistry, but the before-bed meal is quite sneaky. If you absolutely must have something close to bedtime, I recommend a smoothie that combines protein, fibrous veggies, and a few fruits like berries or an apple. See Chapter 11 for some examples.

## STEP 3: EAT THE RIGHT FOODS

This health and fitness thing would certainly be a lot easier if there weren't so many tasty foods out there to indulge in. Who doesn't want to eat all of the time?

I definitely find satisfaction in a good meal, but my wife, Amy, and I have figured out how to create delicious meals that burn fat rather than pack it on. I've included a number of those creations in this book so you don't feel like you're missing out on anything once you get going with this plan. If you've tried a few diets before, you might be expecting the same old tasteless and boring meals that throw together a protein and a vegetable without any flair or flavor. That's not happening here. I want you to enjoy your meals and have an easy time making them as well. I would venture to say that the meals in this book are perhaps the tastiest you'll have ever tried on any "diet."

You can definitely follow your own recipes if you prefer, as long as they meet the criteria that I lay out here. It's simply a matter of what's best for you. However you choose to map out your week of meals, I do suggest that you try two things.

## Nola's Story

"I loved the All-Day Fat-Burning Diet and felt *really* good throughout the entire 21 days. Overall, it was a wonderful experience, and I plan to continue using this plan for another 21 days at least. I have felt good, lost 5 pounds during it, and was definitely looking thinner and leaner using the naked mirror test, as I call it. This has been an incredible learning experience, and I felt very strong and empowered by it. I never thought I could live without bread, but [going without] it hasn't bothered me one bit. Oh, and I just should also mention that my energy throughout the entire program was out of this world! Thank you for a wonderful experience!"

1. **Start your day with protein (whenever that first meal is for you).**

2. **Add more carbohydrates throughout the day.**

I know this may sound completely counterintuitive to what you've been told, especially about carbohydrates. The reason I recommend following these two guidelines is because protein in the morning keeps you full longer, doesn't spike your blood sugar, and keeps you more focused for hours.

The reverse is true if you start with carbs first thing in the morning. Eating a big bowl of cereal or oatmeal, bagel, toast, muffin, or other typical breakfast option is a disaster waiting to happen. These carbs are quickly digested, which then spikes your blood sugar. A "crash" soon follows, leaving you feeling drained and foggy. You then find yourself craving a fix of caffeine or sugar just to make it to lunch.

Adding more protein to your morning meal also allows your natural morning spike of cortisol to occur, which is very important for maintaining healthy circadian rhythms. Normally, cortisol levels are highest in the morning when you wake up (in the presence of light) and lowest at night before going to bed. Anything you do to mess with this natural light-dark cycle will backfire, confuse your hormones, and sabotage your ability to lose fat. On top of that, it turns you into a cranky mess of a person. In studies where this natural circadian rhythm has been purposely disrupted, researchers have noted lowered leptin levels, insulin resistance, inverted cortisol rhythms, and increased blood pressure.[2] These conditions all totally wreck your health and fat-loss efforts.

Even if you decide not to have anything to eat in the morning (which is totally fine if that's what your body is telling you), your cortisol will still stay high because it will be required to break down stored sugar to maintain healthy blood sugar levels. Eating a high-carb breakfast shuts down your morning cortisol response because the surge of ingested sugar tells your body that cortisol is no longer needed to break down fuel. At this time of day, that's the wrong message to be sending to your body. Knowing this, you can approach your morning meal a little more intelligently. Some of the recipes you'll find on your feast days will seem to be high-carb meals; however, these "good carb" meals also contain a considerable amount of protein to get your day started right.

Here are some ideas.

- Gluten-free oatmeal with hemp seeds (protein), peanut butter (protein), ground flaxseeds, and berries

- Veggie omelet

- Morning shake with hemp seeds, almond butter, or protein powder (roughly 30 grams of protein)

- No-grain cereal—berries, chopped nuts, hemp, shredded coconut, almond milk

- Green juice (almost no protein), followed by eggs (protein)

---

## Pheba's Story

No matter what your situation, this program can help you get to a better place.

Consider Pheba. She had already started to make positive changes in her life when she realized her bad eating and lifestyle habits were seriously impacting her health.

"I started changes in my diet back in November 2014 when the doctor told me I had type 2 diabetes. I'd gone to three doctors to find out why I'd been getting insect bite–like hives on my arms one week after another since September. The third doctor ordered labs to be drawn. My blood sugar was 307, and my weight at my heaviest was 205 pounds. Since that time, I cut out 95 percent of refined sugars and carbohydrates. I also tried to be more consistent with exercise. I lost 25 pounds before starting Yuri's program and brought my blood sugar level to the low 100s. Since starting the program, I've lost an additional 10 pounds and have many days that my blood sugar levels are in the 90s. My A1C is now 5.8. I have more energy now and don't crave sweets like I used to. I plan on continuing this as a part of my lifestyle now."

As you progress throughout the day, your cortisol levels will naturally fall as the sun sets and your body gets the message that it's almost bedtime. This is how we humans are built.

It then makes more sense to have a slightly higher-carbohydrate meal because doing so can help keep cortisol levels low. I'm not saying that having pasta and bread before bed is a smart idea, but I am suggesting that having one to two fists of starchy carbs is usually better later in the day than first thing in the morning. As always, it's important to have a well-balanced meal with clean protein, fit fats, and fibrous veggies along with your starchy carb or fruit intake.

Here are simple ideas for a fat-burning, circadian-friendly dinnertime meal.

- Salmon with steamed greens, one fist of mashed sweet potatoes (starchy carbs), and a side salad
- Gluten-free pasta (starchy carbs) with meatballs
- Lentils and brown rice (starchy carbs) with a side salad and/or steamed greens

Even on your Low-Carb Days, do your best to have more of your carbs later in the day.

## THE 5-DAY FOOD-CYCLING FORMULA: A QUICK GUIDE

Note that the following food portions are *per day*.

### *Low-Carb Day*

Protein = 3 palm-size portions (women)/4 palm-size portions (men)

Starchy carbs/fruit = up to ½ fist-size portion

Fibrous veggies = at least 2 hand bowls

Fit fats = 4 thumb-size portions (women)/8 thumb-size portions (men)

### Food Guidelines

Goal = less than 50 grams of net carbs on this day

- Avoid starchy carbs and fruit.
- Eat protein at each meal.
- Make fats your main energy source on this day.
- Eat unlimited amounts of fibrous veggies.
- Eat when you're hungry, and stop when you're full.

### Exercise Guidelines

Do interval speed bursts (5 to 10 minutes), preferably in the morning and/or on an empty stomach, followed by 30 or more minutes of low-intensity cardio (optional).

## 1-Day Feast

Protein = 2 palm-size portions (women)/3 palm-size portions (men)

Starchy carbs/fruit = at least 3 fist-size portions (women)/ 4 fist-size portions (men)

Fibrous veggies = at least 3 hand bowls

Fit fats = 5 thumb-size portions (women)/10 thumb-size portions (men)

### Food Guidelines

Goal = a minimum of 250 grams of net carbohydrates

- Eat healthy feast foods—ad libitum—without feeling guilty.
- Don't binge or stuff yourself; eat until you're 80 percent full, not to the point of discomfort.
- Eat your biggest meal after you work out.
- If you can't eat more at any given meal, then graze throughout the day on nuts, fruit, or other healthy foods.

### Exercise Guidelines

If possible, do your full-body metabolic conditioning workout 1 to 2 hours before you begin your feast day or before your biggest meal of the day.

## 1-Day Fast

Goal = nothing but water and herbal teas for 18 to 24 hours

### Food Guidelines

- Consume nothing but water or herbal tea. It's that simple.
- If you're taking any supplements (multivitamins, fish oil, etc.), give your body a break for this one day.
- Probiotics and digestive enzymes are okay to take since they can provide systemic benefits in the absence of food.

### Exercise Guidelines

- Take the day off and let your body work its magic, or
- Engage in a longer-duration (60 minutes or more) form of very-low-intensity active recovery (such as walking or biking) that will rely on fat as its main fuel source.

## Regular-Cal Day

Protein = 2 palm-size portions (women)/3 palm-size portions (men)

Starchy carbs/fruit = 2 fist-size portions (women)/3 fist-size portions (men)

Fibrous veggies = at least 2 hand bowls

Fit fats = 3 thumb-size portions (women)/6 thumb-size portions (men)

### Food Guidelines

- Eat as you normally would.
- Eat when hungry, and stop when 80 percent full.

### Exercise Guidelines

Do an eccentric strength workout or bodyweight workout on an empty stomach, if possible. Have your biggest meal after you work out.

## Low-Cal Day

Protein = 1 palm-size portion (women)/2 palm-size portions (men)

Starchy carbs/fruit = 1 fist-size portion (women)/2 fist-size portions (men)

Fibrous veggies = at least 2 hand bowls

Fit fats = 3 thumb-size portions (women)/6 thumb-size portions (men)

### Food Guidelines

- Aim to eat about 25 percent less than you did the day before (your Regular-Calorie Day).
- Eat more raw foods and light soups and enjoy smoothies and fresh-pressed green juices, as these food choices are naturally lower in calories.

### Exercise Guidelines

Today is a day off. Let your body relax, recover, and bounce back. If you feel compelled to exercise, then just do some yoga or stretching, go for a long walk, or perform some very light cardio for no more than 30 minutes.

Here's a quick overview of the 21-day plan, including both your workouts and food cycling days.

| DAY 1 | DAY 2 | DAY 3 | DAY 4 | DAY 5 | DAY 6 | DAY 7 |
|---|---|---|---|---|---|---|
| Low Carb Work out | Low Carb Off | 1-Day Feast Work out | 1-Day Fast Off (or active recovery) | Regular Cal Work out | Low Cal Off | Regular Cal Off |

| DAY 8 | DAY 9 | DAY 10 | DAY 11 | DAY 12 | DAY 13 | DAY 14 |
|---|---|---|---|---|---|---|
| Low Carb Sprint | 1-Day Feast Work out | 1-Day Fast Off (or active recovery) | Regular Cal Work out | Low Cal Off | Low Carb Off (or sprint) | 1-Day Feast Work out |

| DAY 15 | DAY 16 | DAY 17 | DAY 18 | DAY 19 | DAY 20 | DAY 21 |
|---|---|---|---|---|---|---|
| 1-Day Fast Off (or active recovery) | Regular Cal Work out | Low Cal Off | Low Carb Sprint | 1-Day Feast Work out | 1-Day Fast Off (or active recovery) | Regular Cal Work out |

# CHAPTER 10

# THE 21-DAY MEAL PLAN AND FAT-BURNING RECIPES

Let me introduce you to the proven 21-day meal plan that has produced the astonishing transformations you've read about throughout this book.

You'll notice that this 21-day plan incorporates roughly four cycles of the 5-Day Food-Cycling Formula (and yes, Days 1 and 2 are both Low-Carb Days—that's not a typo). For best results, I strongly recommend you follow the plan as it's laid out here. However, feel free to swap meals (from similar days) if some of them don't work for you.

Once you've eaten your way through these 21 days, you can repeat the cycle. After all, this is not a diet that you follow for just a few weeks but rather a way of eating that you can live with forever. In Chapter 12, I'll show you a few different options for maintaining this food-cycling program for life. For now, commit to following this proven plan.

*Note:* The recipes begin on page 221, following this outline.

## DAY 1: LOW CARB

**Breakfast:** Veggie Omelet

**Lunch:** Green Protein Salad

**Dinner:** Creamy Tomato Soup with Sausage

## DAY 2: LOW CARB

**Breakfast:** Coco-Berry Blast

**Lunch:** Creamy Kale Salad

**Dinner:** Salmon with Vegetables

## DAY 3: 1-DAY FEAST

**Breakfast:** Green Almond Smoothie

**Lunch:** Quinoa Chili

**Dinner:** Seared Halibut, Peach Salsa, and Cooled Potatoes

## DAY 4: 1-DAY FAST

## DAY 5: REGULAR CAL

**Breakfast:** Garden Green Smoothie

**Lunch:** Southwestern Chicken Salad

**Dinner:** Garlic Shrimp and Brassica

## DAY 6: LOW CAL

**Breakast:** Quinoa, Egg, and Smoked Salmon

**Lunch:** Nori Wraps

**Dinner:** Zucchini Pasta with Marinara Sauce

### DAY 7: REGULAR CAL

**Breakfast:** Chocolate-Covered-Nuts Smoothie

**Lunch:** Nutty Quinoa and Black Bean Salad

**Dinner:** Juicy Steak with Cold Cashew Mayo Potato Salad

### DAY 8: LOW CARB

**Breakfast:** No Oat–Meal

**Lunch:** Broccoli-Kale Soup

**Dinner:** Mexican Shrimp Salad

### DAY 9: 1-DAY FEAST

**Breakfast:** Gluten-Free Banana-Coconut Pancakes

**Lunch:** Salmon Teriyaki Rice Bowl

**Dinner:** Red Lentil Curry–Covered Rice

### DAY 10: 1-DAY FAST

### DAY 11: REGULAR CAL

**Breakfast:** Vanilla Chia Seed Pudding

**Lunch:** Greens, Mango, and Avocado Salad

**Dinner:** Quinoa Veggie Bowl

### DAY 12: LOW CAL

**Breakfast:** Greeny Zingy Smoothie

**Lunch:** Sweet and Savory Kale Salad

**Dinner:** Soothing Squash Salad

## DAY 13: LOW CARB

**Breakfast:** Cauliflower, Meet Eggs

**Lunch:** Green Navy Bowl

**Dinner:** The World's Greatest Burger

## DAY 14: 1-DAY FEAST

**Breakfast:** Protein Lover's Casserole

**Lunch:** Cherry Protein Smoothie

**Dinner:** Choco-Coco-Oatmeal Pancakes

## DAY 15: 1-DAY FAST

## DAY 16: REGULAR CAL

**Breakfast:** Tangy Glowing Green Smoothie

**Lunch:** Sardinian Salad

**Dinner:** Tomato Bean Soup

## DAY 17: LOW CAL

**Breakfast:** Zesty Tropical Green Smoothie

**Lunch:** Thai Salad

**Dinner:** Pesto Zucchini Pasta

## DAY 18: LOW CARB

**Breakfast:** Creamy Avocado Smoothie

**Lunch:** Chicken Lettuce Wraps

**Dinner:** Chicken Breast with Fresh Salsa

## DAY 19: 1-DAY FEAST

**Breakfast:** Strawberry-Vanilla-Oat Shake

**Lunch:** Brown Rice with Steamed Greens, Roasted Veggies, and Avocado

**Dinner:** Mushroom Chicken Pasta

## DAY 20: 1-DAY FAST

## DAY 21: REGULAR CAL

**Breakfast:** Green Apple Cinnamon Smoothie

**Lunch:** Crunchy Green Pear Salad

**Dinner:** Soothing Stew for the Soul

# DAY 1: LOW CARB

# Veggie Omelet

MAKES 1 TO 2 SERVINGS

1 tablespoon butter

½ small onion, chopped

½ bell pepper, chopped

1 cup chopped mushrooms

3 eggs

Sea salt and ground black pepper

1 cup chopped spinach

2 tablespoons chopped fresh basil or 2 teaspoons dried (optional)

**1.** In a medium skillet over medium heat, melt the butter. Cook the onion, bell pepper, and mushrooms for 4 to 5 minutes, stirring occasionally, until the vegetables are just tender.

**2.** While the vegetables are cooking, whisk the eggs together in a bowl and add sea salt and ground black pepper to taste.

**3.** Add the egg mixture to the pan and cook for 1 to 2 minutes, or until the eggs begin to set on the bottom of the pan. Add the spinach and basil, if using. Gently lift the edges of the omelet with a spatula to let the uncooked part of the eggs flow toward the edges and cook. Continue cooking for 2 to 3 minutes, or until the center of the omelet starts to look dry.

**4.** Using a spatula, gently fold one edge of the omelet over the other. Let the omelet cook for another minute, or until it reaches your desired doneness.

**5.** Slide the omelet onto a plate. Cut it in half and serve it with a side of avocado and/or bacon.

# Green Protein Salad

**MAKES 2 TO 3 SERVINGS**

1 tablespoon butter

1 chicken breast, sliced widthwise to create 2 thin halves

1 head lettuce or equivalent amount mixed greens

1 tomato, chopped

1 avocado, cubed

1 orange or yellow bell pepper, chopped

¼ cucumber, peeled and sliced

¼ cup pitted black olives

¼ sweet onion or 1 shallot, sliced

Handful of sprouts (optional)

2 tablespoons olive oil

Juice of ½ lemon

Pinch of sea salt

**1.** In a small skillet over medium heat, melt the butter. Cook the chicken breast halves for 4 to 6 minutes, turning once, or until a thermometer inserted in the thickest portion registers 165°F and the juices run clear. Remove from the heat.

**2.** When cool enough to handle, chop the chicken into cubes or strips.

**3.** In a large bowl, combine the chicken, lettuce or mixed greens, tomato, avocado, bell pepper, cucumber, olives, onion or shallot, and sprouts (if using).

**4.** Top with the olive oil, lemon juice, and sea salt. Toss until evenly coated and serve.

# Creamy Tomato Soup with Sausage

MAKES 3 TO 4 SERVINGS

2 tablespoons butter

1 onion, chopped

2 cloves garlic, minced

1 can (28 ounces) diced tomatoes, undrained

1 cup organic chicken broth

1 cup water

1 cup coconut milk

1 tablespoon paprika

1 tablespoon dried oregano

1 avocado, chopped

1 cooked gluten-free sausage, chopped

2 tablespoons finely chopped cilantro

Salt and ground black pepper

**1.** In a large pot over medium heat, melt the butter. Cook the onion and garlic, stirring frequently, until tender.

**2.** Add the tomatoes with their liquid, the broth, and the water. Bring to a boil, then simmer uncovered for 5 minutes. Add the coconut milk, paprika, and oregano, then turn off the heat and let sit to cool briefly.

**3.** Pour the soup into a blender and puree until smooth (keep the lid open slightly to allow heat to escape).

**4.** Serve in bowls and top with the avocado, sausage, and cilantro. Season to taste with the salt and pepper.

# DAY 2: LOW CARB

## Coco-Berry Blast

**MAKES 2 SERVINGS**

1 cup almond milk
1 cup coconut milk
Handful of fresh spinach
1 cup frozen or fresh berries
1 tablespoon chia seeds

2 tablespoons hemp seeds
1–2 scoops protein powder
(optional)
3 or 4 drops liquid stevia (optional)

In a blender, combine the almond and coconut milk, spinach, berries, chia seeds, hemp seeds, protein powder, and stevia (if using). Blend until smooth.

# Creamy Kale Salad

**MAKES 3 TO 4 SERVINGS**

½ cup tahini

¼ cup water

Juice of 1 lemon

1 clove garlic, minced

2 tablespoons olive oil

Sea salt and ground black pepper

1 head kale or other salad green,
    stemmed and chopped

1 cucumber, peeled and chopped

1 avocado, chopped

1 tomato, chopped

1 can (15 ounces) chickpeas,
    rinsed and drained (optional)

2 tablespoons hemp seeds

**1.** In a large bowl, whisk together the tahini, water, lemon juice, garlic, olive oil, and sea salt and pepper to taste.

**2.** Add the kale, cucumber, avocado, tomato, chickpeas (if using), and hemp seeds. Toss with the dressing until combined and serve.

# Salmon with Vegetables

MAKES 2 SERVINGS

2 salmon fillets

Sea salt and ground black pepper

3 handfuls of spinach, kale, or
Swiss chard

1 tablespoon butter or coconut oil

½ lemon

**1.** Season both sides of the salmon with the sea salt and pepper and let rest for a moment.

**2.** In a steamer, bring some water to a boil over high heat. Turn down the heat, add the greens to the steamer basket, and cover. Steam for 5 minutes, or until tender-crisp.

**3.** Meanwhile, in a medium pan over medium-low heat, melt the butter or coconut oil. Cook the salmon for 6 to 8 minutes, turning once, or until opaque, being careful not to burn either side.

**4.** Serve the salmon alongside the greens. Squeeze some lemon juice over both, and enjoy. You can also have a side salad with your meal.

# DAY 3: 1-DAY FEAST

## Green Almond Smoothie

MAKES 2 TO 3 SERVINGS

Handful of spinach

Handful of chopped, stemmed kale

1 tablespoon almond butter

¼ cup almonds

1 tablespoon hemp seeds

1 tablespoon ground flaxseed

2 cups coconut water

1 cup canned coconut cream

1 teaspoon maple syrup

5 drops liquid stevia

In a blender, combine the spinach, kale, almond butter, almonds, hemp seeds, flaxseed, coconut water, coconut cream, maple syrup, and stevia. Blend until smooth.

# Quinoa Chili

*This is probably the most delicious chili I've tasted, courtesy of my wife, Amy. It has a very "comfort food" feel and is loaded with tons of great nutrition. It's best to prepare it early in the morning so that it's ready for lunch and/or dinner.*

**MAKES 4 TO 6 SERVINGS**

2 tablespoons coconut oil

2½ pounds ground sirloin

2 onions, chopped

6 cloves garlic, minced

1 red bell pepper, chopped

1 orange or yellow bell pepper, chopped

1 can (19 ounces) kidney beans

1 can (15 ounces) black beans

2 cans (14 or 28 ounces each) diced tomatoes

3 tablespoons tomato paste

1 cup quinoa, rinsed

2 cups beef broth

1 tablespoon chili powder

1 teaspoon paprika

1 teaspoon ground cumin

½ teaspoon sea salt

Roasted jalapeño chile peppers, hot sauce, and/or avocado

**1.** In a large pot over medium heat, melt the coconut oil and then cook the beef until no longer pink. Add the onions and cook for 5 minutes. Add the garlic and bell peppers and cook for 5 minutes, stirring occasionally.

**2.** Add the kidney beans, black beans, tomatoes, tomato paste, quinoa, beef broth, chili powder, paprika, cumin, and sea salt. Simmer, partially covered, for 3 hours to let the magic happen, stirring occasionally. (You can eat it after 1 hour, but the longer you leave it, the tastier it gets.)

**3.** Serve in bowls, garnished with the roasted peppers, hot sauce, and/or avocado–they're all delicious!

# Seared Halibut, Peach Salsa, and Cooled Potatoes

MAKES 2 SERVINGS

**Potatoes**

½ pound baby potatoes

**Salsa**

1 peach, chopped
1 red bell pepper, chopped
¼ cup thinly sliced scallions
¼ cup chopped arugula
1 clove garlic, minced
Juice of 1 lemon
2 teaspooons dried oregano

Pinch of sea salt and ground black
   pepper
Pinch of ground red pepper

**Fish**

Juice of ½ lemon
2 tablespoons olive oil
½ teaspoon paprika
1 clove garlic, minced
2 skinless halibut fillets
2 tablespoons butter
Pinch of sea salt and ground black
   pepper

**1.** *To make the potatoes:* Put the potatoes in a medium pot and cover with cold water. Bring to a boil over high heat, reduce the heat to medium, and cover. Gently boil for 20 minutes, or until tender. Refrigerate for several hours to cool.

**2.** *To make the salsa:* In a medium bowl, combine the peach, bell pepper, scallions, arugula, garlic, lemon juice, oregano, salt, black pepper, and red pepper. Toss gently. Let stand for at least 10 to 15 minutes before serving.

**3.** *To make the fish:* In a large glass bowl, whisk together the lemon juice, oil, paprika, and garlic. Add the fish, turning to coat with the marinade. Cover and let stand for 15 minutes.

**4.** In a large pan over medium heat, melt the butter. Remove the fish from the marinade. Discard the leftover marinade. Sprinkle the fish evenly with salt and black pepper and place it in the pan. Sear for 6 minutes, turning once, or until the fish flakes easily.

**5.** Serve the fish alongside the salsa and the cooled potatoes.

# DAY 4: 1-DAY FAST

Water or herbal tea

# DAY 5: REGULAR CAL

## Breakfast

## Garden Green Smoothie

MAKES 2 SERVINGS

Handful of spinach
Handful of stemmed kale
2 tablespoons hemp seeds
1 tablespoon ground flaxseed

1 banana
2 cups water
3 or 4 ice cubes

In a blender, combine the spinach, kale, hemp seeds, flaxseed, banana, water, and ice cubes. Blend until smooth.

# Southwestern Chicken Salad

MAKES 2 SERVINGS

1 teaspoon ground cumin

1 teaspoon paprika

½ teaspoon garlic powder

½ teaspoon chipotle chili powder

¼ teaspoon salt

¼ teaspoon ground cinnamon

1 chicken breast, sliced widthwise to create 2 thin halves

1 tablespoon butter

1 head romaine lettuce, chopped

1 mango, peeled and chopped

½ avocado, chopped

2 tablespoons olive oil (optional)

**1.** In a small bowl, combine the cumin, paprika, garlic powder, chili powder, salt, and cinnamon. Rub the spice mixture onto the chicken breast halves. Let the chicken rest for 5 to 10 minutes, or place it in a resealable plastic bag and refrigerate for several hours before cooking.

**2.** In a skillet over medium heat, melt the butter. Cook the chicken for 4 to 6 minutes, turning once, or until a thermometer inserted in the thickest portion registers 165°F and the juices run clear. Remove from the heat.

**3.** When cool enough to handle, chop the chicken into cubes or strips.

**4.** In a big bowl, combine the romaine, mango, and avocado. Add the chicken, toss it with the olive oil, if using, or a healthy dressing of your choice, and serve.

# Garlic Shrimp and Brassica

**MAKES 2 TO 3 SERVINGS**

2–3 teaspoons butter

1 pound raw medium shrimp, peeled, deveined, tails removed

1 head garlic (yes, indeed), chopped

½ head kale, stemmed and chopped

2 handfuls of Brussels sprouts, trimmed

1 cup baby carrots

Sea salt and ground black pepper

**1.** In a medium skillet over medium heat, melt 1 teaspoon of the butter. Cook the shrimp for 1 minute, stirring frequently. Add the garlic and continue cooking for 3 minutes, or until the shrimp turns opaque. Remove from the heat.

**2.** Meanwhile, in a steamer, steam the kale, Brussels sprouts, and carrots for 5 minutes, or until slightly tender.

**3.** Melt the remaining butter in a separate skillet over medium heat. Add the steamed veggies. Cook, stirring frequently, for 2 minutes. Add sea salt and pepper to taste and serve alongside the shrimp.

# DAY 6: LOW CAL

## Quinoa, Egg, and Smoked Salmon

MAKES 2 SERVINGS

½ cup quinoa

1 tablespoon butter

2 eggs

Pinch of sea salt and ground
black pepper

1 avocado, chopped

2–4 smoked salmon shavings

½ lemon

2 tablespoons sliced scallions

1. Cook the quinoa according to package directions.

2. In a small skillet over medium heat, melt the butter. Add the eggs and prepare as desired. Season with sea salt and pepper.

3. Serve the quinoa topped with the cooked eggs, avocado, and salmon. Drizzle with the juice from the lemon half and top with the scallions.

# Nori Wraps

*You don't need sandwiches when you have wraps that are this good.*

**MAKES 2 SERVINGS**

4 sheets nori

1 avocado, thinly sliced

1 mango, peeled and thinly sliced

1 handful of alfalfa or pea sprouts

¼ cucumber, thinly sliced

Lay out 1 sheet of nori, moisten it with a sprinkle of water, and place one-quarter of the avocado, mango, sprouts, and cucumber on it. Roll up into a wrap. Repeat with the remaining ingredients.

# Zucchini Pasta with Marinara Sauce

*This is one of my all-time-favorite no-cook pastas. It's gluten free, light, and loaded with flavor.*

**MAKES 2 SERVINGS**

1 zucchini, peeled

2 cloves garlic, minced

1 cup sun-dried tomatoes

3 cups chopped tomatoes

2 dates, pitted and soaked in water

¼ red onion, chopped

2 tablespoons olive oil

½ handful of chopped fresh parsley

½ handful of fresh basil

⅓ cup pitted black olives (optional)

Pinch of sea salt or kelp/dulse flakes

**1.** Using a vegetable peeler or spiralizer, shave the zucchini into paper-thin "noodles."

**2.** In a food processor, combine the garlic, tomatoes, dates, onion, oil, parsley, basil, olives (if using), and salt or kelp/dulse flakes. Pulse until smooth to create the marinara sauce.

**3.** Plate the zucchini noodles, top with the marinara sauce, and serve.

# DAY 7: REGULAR CAL

## Chocolate-Covered-Nuts Smoothie

**MAKES 2 SERVINGS**

1 cup almond milk

1 cup canned coconut milk

2 tablespoons almond butter

1 tablespoon hemp seeds

1 tablespoon chia seeds

1 tablespoon flax oil

1 tablespoon cacao powder

¼ cup gluten-free rolled oats

1–2 scoops protein powder
(optional)

5–10 drops liquid stevia

In a blender, combine the almond milk, coconut milk, almond butter, hemp seeds, chia seeds, oil, cacao powder, oats, protein powder (if using), and stevia. Blend until smooth.

# Nutty Quinoa and Black Bean Salad

*This is a great salad that can be enjoyed warm or cold. Store leftovers in the fridge and enjoy the next day if you like.*

**MAKES 2 TO 3 SERVINGS**

1 cup quinoa

Sea salt

¼ cup canned black beans, rinsed and drained

2 tablespoons pine nuts

½ bell pepper, chopped

¼ red onion, chopped

10 olives, pitted and chopped

6 small cherry tomatoes, halved

½ handful of chopped cilantro

Ground black pepper

2 tablespoons olive oil

1 tablespoon apple cider vinegar or lemon juice

**1.** In a medium pot over medium-high heat, cook the quinoa with the sea salt according to package directions.

**2.** Taste the grain. There should be just a little resistance, and the opaque spiraled ring of the germ should show. If necessary, continue cooking until done. Then, add the black beans if you'd like them warmed.

**3.** Meanwhile, in a small pan over medium heat, lightly toast the pine nuts for 3 minutes, or until they turn golden brown in spots. Watch carefully so you don't burn them! Place them in a salad bowl.

**4.** Add the quinoa, black beans, bell pepper, onion, olives, tomatoes, cilantro, and salt and black pepper to the salad bowl. Stir in the olive oil and vinegar or lemon juice. Give it a toss and enjoy.

# Juicy Steak with Cold Cashew Mayo Potato Salad

*Enjoy a palm-size portion of delicious steak (ideally, grass fed) along with a unique potato salad that is actually good for your gut and weight-loss efforts. Since the potatoes are cooked, then cooled, they retain a high amount of their resistant starch—a very helpful fiber for gut health and weight loss.*

**MAKES 2 SERVINGS**

### Steak

2 palm-size steaks (or 1 larger steak, cut in half)

1 whole + 1 minced clove garlic

Sea salt and ground black pepper

1 teaspoon chopped fresh thyme

1 teaspoon chopped fresh rosemary

1 tablespoon coconut aminos

8–10 small golden potatoes

2 tablespoons butter

### Cashew Mayo

1 tablespoon apple cider vinegar

3 tablespoons lemon juice

1 cup cashews

½ cup water

1 teaspoon chopped fresh thyme

Sea salt and ground black pepper

¼ cup chopped chives

**1.** *To marinate the steak:* In a bowl, rub both sides of the steaks with the whole garlic. Mix together the sea salt, pepper, thyme, and rosemary, and rub the steaks with this herb mixture. Add the coconut aminos. Let sit in the bowl for 15 minutes (or refrigerate for several hours if you want a better marinade).

**2.** Meanwhile, bring a medium pot of salted water to a boil and add the potatoes. Cook for 5 to 8 minutes, or until tender—you should be able to put a fork in the potatoes without breaking them apart. Strain the potatoes and cover with ice-cold water for 2 minutes. Drain, then set aside or place in the fridge to cool.

**3.** When the potatoes have cooled, slice them in half and add them to a salad bowl.

**4.** *To make the cashew mayo:* In a blender, combine the vinegar, lemon juice, cashews, water, thyme, and sea salt and pepper to taste. Blend until smooth. Pour over the potatoes. Mix well and garnish with the chives. Set aside.

**5.** *To cook the steak:* Heat a medium pan over medium heat. Warm the butter, minced garlic, and steak marinade mixture.

**6.** Add the steaks to the pan and cook for 4 to 6 minutes, turning once, or until a thermometer inserted in the center registers 145°F for medium-rare. Let stand for 10 minutes before serving.

**7.** To serve, drizzle the remaining butter/marinade mixture from the pan over the steaks. Serve alongside the potato salad, with steamed greens or a small green salad.

*Note:* Since some people experience gas and bloating when incorporating more resistant starch into their diets, stick to a handful-size (1-cup) serving of the potatoes, at least your first time around.

# DAY 8: LOW CARB

## No Oat–Meal

**MAKES 1 SERVING**

¼ cup chia seeds

¼ cup shredded unsweetened coconut

¼ cup hemp seeds

¼ cup chopped almonds

2 tablespoons ground flaxseed

1 tablespoon ground cinnamon

1 cup hot water

2 or 3 drops liquid stevia (optional)

2 tablespoons unsweetened coconut milk

1 small apple, finely chopped (optional)

**1.** In a bowl, combine the chia seeds, coconut, hemp seeds, almonds, flax-seed, and cinnamon.

**2.** Pour the hot water over the mixture and let sit for 3 to 5 minutes.

**3.** Add the stevia (if using) and coconut milk to the bowl and stir to combine.

**4.** Top with the chopped apple (or not, if you want to keep your carb count even lower) and enjoy.

# Broccoli-Kale Soup

**MAKES 2 TO 3 SERVINGS**

1 tablespoon butter

4 cloves garlic, minced

1 onion, chopped

1 cup chopped carrots

2 ribs celery, chopped

2 heads broccoli, chopped

1 bunch kale, stemmed

1 quart vegetable broth

**1.** In a large pot over medium heat, melt the butter and cook the garlic, onion, carrots, and celery until lightly browned.

**2.** Add the broccoli and kale.

**3.** Pour in the vegetable broth and bring to a boil. Lower the heat, cover, and simmer for 45 minutes, or until the vegetables are soft.

**4.** Cool the soup slightly, then pour it into a blender. Puree and enjoy!

# Mexican Shrimp Salad

*I have no idea if this is an actual Mexican dish—I don't think it is—but the flavors are certainly authentic. You'll love this quick and delicious meal.*

**MAKES 2 SERVINGS**

2 tablespoons butter

1 pound raw medium shrimp, peeled, deveined, tails removed

2 cloves garlic, minced

Juice of 1 lime

2 tablespoons olive oil

Small handful of chopped cilantro

½ teaspoon chili powder

2 handfuls of chopped baby spinach or baby kale

1 ripe avocado, cubed

½ cup cherry tomatoes (optional)

Sea salt and ground black pepper

**1.** In a medium skillet over medium heat, melt the butter. Cook the shrimp for 1 minute. Add the garlic and cook, stirring frequently, for 3 minutes, or until the shrimp turns opaque.

**2.** In a bowl, combine the shrimp with the lime juice, olive oil, cilantro, and chili powder and let marinate for 5 minutes.

**3.** Add the spinach or kale, avocado, and tomatoes (if using). Season to taste with salt and pepper, mix well, and serve.

# DAY 9: 1-DAY FEAST

## Gluten-Free Banana-Coconut Pancakes

*These pancakes are not only gluten-free but vegan. Add some protein by having 3 pieces of bacon or some shaved ham.*

MAKES 2 SERVINGS

**Egg Substitute (see note)**

1 tablespoon chia seeds

1 tablespoon ground flaxseed

¼ cup hot or boiling water

**Gluten-Free Flour**

1½ cups millet flour

1½ cups almond flour

1 cup quinoa flour

1 cup buckwheat flour

2 cups tapioca flour

**Pancakes**

1¼ cups Gluten-Free Flour

2 teaspoons baking powder

¼ teaspoon salt

1 scoop protein powder (optional)

1¼ cups almond milk

Egg Substitute or 2 eggs

3 tablespoons coconut oil, melted

¼ cup unsweetened shredded coconut + additional for garnish

½ teaspoon ground cinnamon

1 banana, chopped + additional slices for garnish

Maple syrup

**1.** *To make the egg substitute:* In a small bowl, mix together the chia seeds, flaxseed, and water. Set aside for 10 minutes.

**2.** *To make the gluten-free flour:* In a large bowl, stir together the millet, almond, quinoa, buckwheat, and tapioca flours until evenly blended.

**3.** *To make the pancakes:* In a separate large bowl, combine 1¼ cups of the Gluten-Free Flour, the baking powder, salt, and protein powder (if using). Add the almond milk, Egg Substitute, and coconut oil and mix well. Add the coconut, cinnamon, and chopped banana and mix well.

**4.** In a large skillet over medium heat, use half the batter to cook 3 pancakes, turning them once. Repeat with the remaining batter. Garnish the pancakes with additional coconut and banana slices and serve with the maple syrup.

*Note:* Or use 2 eggs, but the pancakes will not be vegan.

# Salmon Teriyaki Rice Bowl

**MAKES 2 SERVINGS**

1 teaspoon sesame oil

2 tablespoons coconut aminos

1 clove garlic, minced

1" piece fresh ginger, peeled and grated

1 tablespoon honey

1 cup brown rice

2 handfuls of baby spinach, Swiss chard, or kale (stemmed)

2 small wild-caught salmon fillets

1 tablespoon coconut oil

1 avocado, sliced (optional)

1 tablespoon sesame seeds

**1.** In a small saucepan over high heat, bring the sesame oil, coconut aminos, garlic, ginger, and honey to a gentle boil. Lower the heat and simmer, uncovered, until slightly thickened, 5 to 10 minutes.

**2.** Meanwhile, cook the rice according to package directions and steam the spinach, chard, or kale.

**3.** Brush both sides of the salmon with the reduced marinade and let sit for a moment.

**4.** In a medium pan over medium-low heat, melt the coconut oil. Cook the marinated salmon fillets for 6 to 8 minutes, turning once, or until the fish is opaque.

**5.** Place the rice, steamed greens, and avocado slices (if using) in 2 bowls. Top with the salmon and remaining marinade from the pan. Sprinkle the sesame seeds over the top and enjoy.

# Red Lentil Curry–Covered Rice

*This is a nice, hearty dish. It can be enjoyed on Regular-Cal Days, Low-Cal Days, and feast days, just in varying portions.*

MAKES 2 TO 3 SERVINGS

1 cup brown rice

3½ cups low-sodium vegetable
broth, divided

1 cup red lentils

2 tablespoons coconut oil

1 onion, chopped

2 cloves garlic, minced

4 medium carrots, chopped

1 can (14 ounces) tomato paste

¼ cup water

1" piece fresh ginger, peeled and
grated

1 tablespoon curry powder

1 teaspoon turmeric powder

½ teaspoon garam masala

Sea salt and ground black pepper

¼ cup canned coconut milk

2 or 3 sprigs cilantro

**1.** In a medium saucepan, cover the brown rice with 2 cups of the vegetable broth and bring to a boil. Reduce the heat to low, cover, and cook for 15 to 20 minutes, or until the rice is just tender.

**2.** Meanwhile, in a small saucepan, combine the lentils with the remaining 1½ cups vegetable broth and bring to a boil. Lower the heat and simmer gently for 20 to 30 minutes, uncovered, or until the lentils are tender. Add water if the lentils get too dry before they are fully cooked.

**3.** While the lentils cook, melt the coconut oil in a large skillet over medium heat. Cook the onion, garlic, and carrots for a few minutes, stirring frequently, until fragrant and golden. Add the tomato paste, water, ginger, curry powder, turmeric, garam masala, and sea salt and pepper to taste. Stir and simmer until smooth.

**4.** Add the cooked lentils and coconut milk. Stir to combine and simmer for 5 to 10 minutes. Remove from the heat and serve over the brown rice, garnished with the cilantro sprigs.

# DAY 10: 1-DAY FAST

Water or herbal tea

# DAY 11: REGULAR CAL

## Vanilla Chia Seed Pudding

*This filling pudding will keep you fueled and going for hours. For ultimate convenience, make this the night before so it's ready to go for you in the morning.*

**MAKES 2 SERVINGS**

2 cups almond milk

3 or 4 drops liquid stevia

2 vanilla beans, scraped, or
    1 tablespoon vanilla extract

⅓ cup chia seeds

½ cup blueberries

**1.** In a blender, pulse the almond milk, stevia, and vanilla. Add the chia seeds and pulse one more time.

**2.** Pour the pudding into a bowl and refrigerate for 1 hour, stirring occasionally to keep the chia seeds from sticking together.

**3.** Top with the blueberries and serve.

# Greens, Mango, and Avocado Salad

MAKES 2 SERVINGS

2 handfuls of mixed salad greens

1 avocado, chopped

1 mango, chopped

¼ red onion, chopped

½ handful of chopped cilantro

2 tablespoons olive oil

1 tablespoon apple cider vinegar

Juice of ½ lemon

Sea salt and ground black pepper

**1.** In a large bowl, place the greens, avocado, mango, onion, and cilantro.

**2.** In a small bowl, whisk together the oil, vinegar, lemon juice, and sea salt and pepper to taste.

**3.** Pour the dressing over the salad, toss, and serve.

# Quinoa Veggie Bowl

**MAKES 2 TO 3 SERVINGS**

1 cup quinoa

1 sweet potato, peeled and sliced

1 zucchini, sliced

1 eggplant, sliced

3–4 tablespoons olive oil + additional for serving

½ teaspoon kelp seasoning or sea salt + additional for serving

¼ teaspoon ground black pepper + additional for serving

½ head Swiss chard, kale, or spinach, stemmed

1 avocado, sliced

**1.** Preheat the oven to 350°F. Meanwhile, cook the quinoa according to package directions.

**2.** In a 13" x 9" glass baking dish, place the sweet potato, zucchini, and eggplant slices. Sprinkle with 3 to 4 tablespoons of olive oil, ½ teaspoon of the kelp seasoning or sea salt, and 1 teaspoon of the pepper. Bake for 20 to 30 minutes, or until just tender.

**3.** Meanwhile, steam the Swiss chard, kale, or spinach for 15 to 20 minutes, or until tender.

**4.** In a bowl, serve the quinoa topped with the greens, roasted veggies, and sliced avocado. Add additional olive oil, kelp seasoning or sea salt, and pepper to taste.

# DAY 12: LOW CAL

## Greeny Zingy Smoothie

**MAKES 2 SERVINGS**

1 handful of kale, Swiss chard, or spinach, stemmed

1 small cucumber, peeled and chopped

1 apple, chopped

2 tablespoons hemp seeds

Juice of ¼ lemon

½ tablespoon coconut oil

1 tablespoon Yuri Elkaim's Energy Greens (optional)

½ tablespoon maple syrup, or to taste

4 or 5 ice cubes

2 cups water

1" piece fresh ginger, peeled and grated, juice reserved

In a blender, combine the kale, chard, or spinach with the cucumber, apple, hemp seeds, lemon juice, coconut oil, Energy Greens (if using), maple syrup, ice cubes, and water. Squeeze the juice from the grated ginger into the blender and discard the pulp. Blend until smooth.

# Sweet and Savory Kale Salad

**MAKES 2 SERVINGS**

### Salad

1 handful of kale, stemmed and chopped

2 handfuls of salad greens

1 carrot, cut into matchsticks

¼ head red cabbage, shredded

1 green apple, sliced

¼ cup thinly sliced red onion

¼ cup chopped walnuts

¼ cup canned navy beans, rinsed and drained

### Dressing

3 tablespoons olive oil

Juice of ½ lemon

1 teaspoon apple cider vinegar (optional)

1 teaspoon honey

Sea salt and ground black pepper

**1.** *To make the salad:* In a large bowl, combine the kale, greens, carrot, cabbage, apple, onion, walnuts, and beans.

**2.** *To make the dressing:* In a small bowl, whisk together the oil, lemon juice, vinegar (if using), honey, and sea salt and pepper to taste.

**3.** Pour the dressing over the salad, toss well, and enjoy.

# Soothing Squash Salad

MAKES 2 TO 3 SERVINGS

### Salad

2 cups cubed butternut squash

½ cup canned chickpeas, rinsed and drained

1 cup pecans

2 tablespoons olive oil

1 tablespoon maple syrup

2 handfuls of mixed salad greens

2 tablespoons organic dried cranberries

2 tablespoons crumbled goat cheese (optional)

2 scallions, sliced

### Dressing

2 tablespoons olive oil

1 teaspoon whole grain or Dijon mustard

1 tablespoon maple syrup

Juice of ½ lemon

1 tablespoon ground cinnamon

1 teaspoon ground cumin

Sea salt and ground black pepper

**1.** *To make the salad:* Preheat the oven to 400°F. Line a rimmed baking sheet with parchment paper.

**2.** In a medium bowl, combine the squash, chickpeas, pecans, oil, and maple syrup. Spread the squash mixture on the baking sheet and roast for 25 to 30 minutes, or until the squash is tender but not mushy. Remove from the oven and let cool.

**3.** Assemble the salad in a large bowl by topping the greens with the squash mixture, cranberries, goat cheese (if using), and scallions.

**4.** *To make the dressing:* In a small bowl, whisk together the oil, mustard, maple syrup, lemon juice, cinnamon, cumin, and sea salt and pepper to taste. Drizzle the dressing over the salad, toss well, and serve.

# DAY 13: LOW CARB

## Cauliflower, Meet Eggs

MAKES 2 SERVINGS

2 tablespoons coconut oil

½ head cauliflower, finely chopped

1 onion, chopped

¼ teaspoon paprika

Pinch of sea salt and ground black pepper

3 tablespoons water

2 eggs

1 clove garlic, minced

Juice of ¼ lemon

3 tablespoons finely chopped parsley

1 tablespoon olive oil

**1.** In a large skillet over medium-high heat, heat the coconut oil. Cook the cauliflower and onion for 2 to 3 minutes.

**2.** Add the paprika, sea salt and pepper, and water. Cover the skillet and cook for 3 to 5 minutes, or until the cauliflower is fork-tender but not mushy and has taken on a golden color.

**3.** Meanwhile, in a small skillet, cook 2 eggs the way you like them (over easy, sunny side up, etc.).

**4.** Reduce the heat under the large skillet to low, add the garlic, and cook for 2 minutes, uncovered, stirring constantly. Stir in the lemon juice and cook until evaporated, about 30 seconds.

**5.** To serve, divide the cauliflower mixture between 2 plates. Sprinkle the parsley on top, top with the cooked eggs (and some bacon or sausage if you like), and drizzle with the olive oil.

# Green Navy Bowl

*This bowl is a slight exception on the Low-Carb Day since each serving features ¼ cup of navy beans, which provide about 12 grams of good carbohydrates. Yet you'll still be well below your 50-gram target by the end of the day.*

**MAKES 2 SERVINGS**

½ cup canned navy beans, rinsed and drained

½ cup water

Pinch of sea salt

1 tablespoon curry powder or ground turmeric

2–3 stalks Swiss chard, chopped

1 handful of baby spinach

1 tablespoon sesame seeds

2 tablespoons chopped almonds

1 tablespoon olive oil

Juice of ½ lemon

Ground black pepper

**1.** Warm a small pot over medium heat. Add the beans, water, sea salt, and curry powder or turmeric. Allow the beans to absorb the spices. In so doing, they should take on a yellow tint.

**2.** Meanwhile, steam the Swiss chard and spinach to your desired softness.

**3.** Place the navy beans in a bowl and top them with the steamed greens. Sprinkle with the sesame seeds and almonds.

**4.** Drizzle the olive oil and lemon juice over the top, and season to taste with the pepper.

# The World's Greatest Burger

*We've created the world's best burger, and it's easier to make than you'd think. Seriously. It all starts with good meat. Most burgers get it all wrong by adding a bunch of unnecessary ingredients. This burger is simple and amazingly good. More good news: You can enjoy this burger without the bun, which is perfect for a healthy Low-Carb Day. I would suggest making a basic green salad to accompany your burger.*

**MAKES 2 SERVINGS**

¾ pound finely ground sirloin
Sea salt and ground black pepper
½ tomato, sliced

¼ red onion, sliced
2 pickles, sliced

**1.** Use your clean hands to thoroughly work the meat, then take 1 large handful of meat, roll it into a ball (about the size of a baseball), and flatten it to about a 1" thickness. Repeat to create 1 more burger.

**2.** Season the meat with sea salt and pepper.

**3.** Meanwhile, heat a pan over medium-low heat. Cook the burgers for 4 to 6 minutes, turning once, or until a thermometer inserted in the center registers 160°F and the meat is no longer pink.

**4.** Serve the burgers topped with the sliced tomato, onion, and pickles.

# DAY 14: 1-DAY FEAST

## Protein Lover's Casserole

MAKES 4 SERVINGS

1 sweet potato, peeled

1 red bell pepper, halved and seeded

1 medium yellow squash, peeled

1 medium zucchini, peeled

1 tablespoon coconut oil

½ pound pork or turkey sausages, chopped

¼ cup finely chopped scallions

4 eggs

Sea salt and ground black pepper

**1.** Preheat the oven to 350°F. Either by hand or with a food processor, cut the sweet potato, bell pepper, yellow squash, and zucchini into matchsticks.

**2.** In a medium skillet over medium heat, melt the oil. Add the sausages and cook for 10 minutes, or until no longer pink. Add the sweet potato, bell pepper, yellow squash, and zucchini and cook, stirring frequently, for 10 minutes, or until tender.

**3.** Fill a 13" x 9" baking dish with the meat and vegetable mixture. Sprinkle with the scallions.

**4.** In a medium bowl, whisk the eggs. Pour them over the top of the casserole. Season to taste with sea salt and black pepper. Bake for 25 minutes, or until the center of the casserole is cooked through.

# Cherry Protein Smoothie

MAKES 2 SERVINGS

1 cup frozen cherries

¼ cup almonds

½ cup coconut milk

2 cups almond milk

2 tablespoons hemp seeds

1 tablespoon ground flaxseed

1 scoop vanilla protein powder

In a blender, combine the cherries, almonds, coconut and almond milk, hemp seeds, flaxseed, and protein powder. Blend until smooth and serve.

# Choco-Coco-Oatmeal Pancakes

**MAKES 8 (2 TO 3 SERVINGS)**

2 ripe bananas

2 eggs (or 3 tablespoons ground chia seeds and 9 tablespoons water)

1 cup gluten-free oats

½ cup almond flour

½ cup buckwheat flour

¼ cup tapioca starch

1 scoop vanilla protein powder (optional)

¼ cup unsweetened shredded coconut

¼ cup Enjoy Life semisweet chocolate chips

2 teaspoons baking powder

2 tablespoons ground flaxseed

1 teaspoon vanilla extract

2 tablespoons almond butter

2 tablespoons coconut oil, melted

6 tablespoons almond milk

Pinch of sea salt

Maple syrup

**1.** In a large bowl, mash the bananas with a fork. Add the eggs (or egg substitute) and whisk until well combined.

**2.** Add the oats, flours, tapioca starch, protein powder (if using), coconut, chocolate chips, baking powder, flaxseed, vanilla, almond butter, oil, almond milk, and sea salt. Mix well.

**3.** Lightly butter or oil a large skillet and place it over medium heat. Scoop ¼-cup portions of the pancake batter into the skillet. Cook the pancakes for 4 to 8 minutes, turning once, or until golden brown.

**4.** Serve the pancakes plain or with a small drizzle of maple syrup and a side of bacon or shaved ham.

# DAY 15: 1-DAY FAST

Water or herbal tea

# DAY 16: REGULAR CAL

## Tangy Glowing Green Smoothie

**MAKES 2 SERVINGS**

4 handfuls of spinach or kale
2 tablespoons hemp seeds
½ cucumber
Juice of 1 lime

Juice of 1 lemon
1 cup water
3 or 4 ice cubes

In a blender, combine the spinach or kale, hemp seeds, cucumber, lime juice, lemon juice, water, and ice cubes. Blend until smooth.

# Sardinian Salad

MAKES 2 SERVINGS

### Salad

6 cups salad greens and/or baby
    spinach
1 can (3.75 ounces) sardines or
    anchovies, chopped
1 carrot, grated
¼ fennel bulb, grated
1 cup cherry tomatoes
¼ cup chopped sun-dried tomatoes
¼ red onion, chopped
1 avocado, cubed
¼ cup pitted and chopped black
    olives

### Dressing

3 tablespoons olive oil
Juice of ½ lemon
1 clove garlic, crushed and minced
Sea salt and ground black pepper

**1.** *To make the salad:* In a large salad bowl, combine the greens, sardines or anchovies, carrot, fennel, tomatoes, onion, avocado, and olives.

**2.** *To make the dressing:* In a small bowl, whisk together the oil, lemon juice, garlic, and sea salt and pepper to taste. Drizzle over the salad, toss, and enjoy.

# Tomato Bean Soup

MAKES 4 TO 6 SERVINGS

2 teaspoons coconut oil

1 onion, chopped

3 cloves garlic, minced

3 tablespoons chopped fresh basil or 1 tablespoon dried

½ teaspoon dried thyme

3 cups water

3 cups organic vegetable broth

1 can (15 ounces) organic diced tomatoes

1 can (15 ounces) chickpeas or white beans, rinsed and drained

2 cups chopped kale

2 cups chopped green or red cabbage

1 zucchini, chopped

Pinch of ground red pepper

**1.** In a large pot over medium heat, melt the coconut oil. Cook the onion, stirring frequently, until softened. Add the garlic, basil, and thyme and cook, stirring, for 1 minute.

**2.** Add the water and vegetable broth, tomatoes (with juice), chickpeas or beans, kale, cabbage, zucchini, and ground red pepper. Simmer for 15 minutes, or until the zucchini is soft. Turn off the heat and let rest for a few minutes before serving.

# DAY 17: LOW CAL

## Zesty Tropical Green Smoothie

**MAKES 2 TO 3 SERVINGS**

2 cups coconut water

1 apple, coarsely chopped

1 pear, coarsely chopped

½ cucumber, peeled and chopped

1 handful of spinach

½ avocado

2 ribs celery

2 tablespoons hemp seeds

1 tablespoon ground flaxseed

1" piece fresh ginger, peeled and grated

Juice of ½ lemon

Juice of ½ lime

3–5 drops liquid stevia (optional)

In a blender, combine the coconut water, apple, pear, cucumber, spinach, avocado, celery, hemp seeds, flaxseed, ginger, lemon juice, lime juice, and stevia (if using). Blend until smooth.

# Thai Salad

*This is a delicious salad that will wow your tastebuds. The recipe makes a lot so you can enjoy the leftovers for up to 2 days if they're kept in the fridge.*

MAKES 6 SERVINGS

### Dressing

½ cup peanut butter

3 tablespoons coconut aminos

2 cloves garlic

2 tablespoons lime juice

1 tablespoon roasted sesame oil

2 tablespoons honey

1 tablespoon ginger juice (squeeze peeled, grated fresh ginger over a bowl until you have enough juice)

### Salad

¼ head red cabbage, shredded

3 carrots, shredded

1 head Swiss chard, thinly sliced

1 red bell pepper, thinly sliced

1 yellow bell pepper, thinly sliced

½ cup finely chopped cilantro

½ cup peanuts, coarsely chopped

¼ cup chopped scallions

**1.** *To make the dressing:* In a blender, combine the peanut butter, coconut aminos, garlic, lime juice, oil, honey, and ginger juice. Blend until smooth.

**2.** *To make the salad:* In a large bowl, combine the cabbage, carrots, chard, bell peppers, and cilantro.

**3.** Drizzle the dressing over the salad and toss. Garnish with the peanuts and scallions before serving.

# Pesto Zucchini Pasta

**MAKES 2 SERVINGS**

2 zucchini, peeled

2 cloves garlic

1 cup fresh basil

½ cup pine nuts

2 tablespoons flax oil

2 tablespoons olive oil

2 tablespoons lemon juice

**1.** Using a vegetable peeler or spiralizer, shave the zucchini into "noodles." Place them in a serving bowl.

**2.** In a food processor or blender, combine the garlic, basil, nuts, oils, and lemon juice. Blend well.

**3.** Pour the pesto over the zucchini noodles. Mix well.

# DAY 18: LOW CARB

## Creamy Avocado Smoothie

MAKES 2 SERVINGS

1 avocado, halved, pitted, and peeled

1 handful of baby spinach

2 scoops vanilla protein powder

1 cup unsweetened coconut milk

1 cup almond milk

1 tablespoon Yuri Elkaim's Energy Greens (optional but recommended)

3 or 4 drops liquid stevia

In a blender, combine the avocado, spinach, protein powder, coconut milk, almond milk, Energy Greens (if using), and stevia. Blend until smooth.

# Chicken Lettuce Wraps

**MAKES 4 (2 SERVINGS)**

3 tablespoons coconut oil, divided

2 boneless, skinless chicken
    breasts or thighs, chopped

Sea salt and ground black pepper

Juice of 1 lemon

¼ cup coconut aminos

1 teaspoon chili powder

1 teaspoon sesame oil

2 scallions, finely chopped

1 handful of chopped cilantro

1 cup chopped shiitake mushrooms

½ onion, chopped

3 cloves garlic, minced

1 head iceberg lettuce

1 avocado, sliced

1. In a large pan over medium heat, melt 2 tablespoons of the coconut oil.

2. Add the chicken and season it with sea salt and pepper. Cook for 6 to 8 minutes, turning once, or until no longer pink.

3. In a bowl, combine the lemon juice, coconut aminos, chili powder, sesame oil, scallions, and cilantro. Add the chicken and toss to combine.

4. Add the remaining 1 tablespoon coconut oil to the pan. Cook the mushrooms, onion, and garlic, stirring frequently, for 10 minutes, or until golden. Add to the bowl. Toss to coat.

5. Remove the stem of your lettuce head with a knife and slice the head in half lengthwise. Peel the lettuce into 4 individual "cups" and wash them.

6. Pile the chicken mixture into your lettuce cups, top with avocado, and enjoy!

# Chicken Breast with Fresh Salsa

MAKES 2 SERVINGS

## Salsa

1 avocado, cubed
1 tomato, chopped
¼ red onion, chopped
Small handful of cilantro, chopped
1 tablespoon olive oil
Juice of ¼ lemon

## Chicken

1 clove garlic
1 large chicken breast, sliced widthwise to create 2 thin halves
Pinch of sea salt and ground black pepper
1 tablespoon butter

1. *To make the salsa:* In a bowl, mix together the avocado, tomato, red onion, cilantro, olive oil, and lemon juice. Set aside.

2. *To make the chicken:* Rub the garlic clove over both sides of the chicken breast halves, then season them with sea salt and pepper.

3. In a medium skillet over medium heat, melt the butter. Cook the chicken breast halves for 4 to 6 minutes, turning once, or until a thermometer inserted in the thickest portion registers 165°F and the juices run clear. Remove from the heat.

4. Serve the chicken topped with the fresh salsa. Add sea salt and pepper to taste.

# DAY 19: 1-DAY FEAST

## Strawberry-Vanilla-Oat Shake

MAKES 2 SERVINGS

1 cup frozen or fresh strawberries

½ cup gluten-free oats

½ cup cashews

2 tablespoons hemp seeds

1 cup almond milk

1 cup water or coconut water

1 scoop vanilla protein powder (optional)

1 tablespoon ground flaxseed

1 tablespoon flax oil

1 tablespoon vanilla extract

1 tablespoon ground cinnamon

5–8 drops liquid stevia

In a blender, combine the strawberries, oats, cashews, hemp seeds, almond milk, water, protein powder (if using), flaxseed, oil, vanilla, cinnamon, and stevia. Blend until smooth and serve.

# Brown Rice with Steamed Greens, Roasted Veggies, and Avocado

**MAKES 2 TO 3 SERVINGS**

1 cup brown basmati rice

1 sweet potato, peeled and sliced

1 zucchini, sliced

1 eggplant, sliced

2–3 tablespoons olive oil + additional for serving

Sea salt and ground black pepper

½ head Swiss chard, stemmed

½ head kale, stemmed

1 handful spinach

1 avocado, sliced

Juice of ½ lemon

**1.** Cook the rice according to package directions.

**2.** Preheat the oven to 350°F. In a 13" x 9" glass baking dish, place the sweet potato, zucchini, and eggplant slices and sprinkle them with the olive oil, sea salt, and pepper. Bake for 20 to 30 minutes, or until tender but not mushy.

**3.** Steam the Swiss chard, kale, and spinach for 15 to 20 minutes, or until slightly softened.

**4.** Serve the rice in a bowl, topped with the greens, roasted veggies, and avocado. Add additional olive oil, the lemon juice, and sea salt and pepper to taste.

# Mushroom Chicken Pasta

MAKES 4 SERVINGS

1 pound boneless, skinless chicken breasts

2 tablespoons coconut oil

Sea salt and ground black pepper

1 package (8.8 ounces) organic black rice noodles

1 onion, chopped

8 ounces white or brown mushrooms, sliced

4 cloves garlic, minced

½ cup coconut cream (the solid mass in a can of full-fat coconut milk)

½ cup chicken stock

2 tablespoons lemon juice

1 tablespoon all-purpose gluten-free flour (such as Bob's Red Mill)

¼ cup chopped fresh basil

**1.** Cut the chicken into thumb-size strips. In a large skillet over medium heat, melt the coconut oil. Add the chicken strips, liberally season them with sea salt and pepper, and cook, stirring frequently, for 4 to 5 minutes, or until no longer pink and the juices run clear.

**2.** Remove the chicken from the pan and place it in a bowl. Meanwhile, cook the rice noodles according to package directions, until al dente.

**3.** Add the onion and mushrooms to the skillet and cook, stirring frequently, for 10 minutes. Add the garlic and cook, stirring frequently, for 2 minutes.

**4.** Add the coconut cream, chicken stock, and lemon juice to the skillet. Bring to a boil over high heat. Reduce the heat to medium and add the flour. Stir with a whisk to thoroughly combine.

**5.** Add the chicken back to the skillet and season with sea salt and pepper to taste. Turn off the heat and stir in the noodles.

**6.** Transfer to a serving dish and sprinkle with the fresh basil.

# DAY 20: 1-DAY FAST

Water or herbal tea

# DAY 21: REGULAR CAL

## Green Apple Cinnamon Smoothie

MAKES 2 SERVINGS

2 handfuls of baby spinach

1 apple, peeled, cored, and chopped

2 kiwifruits, peeled and sliced

1 tablespoon ground flaxseed

1 tablespoon hemp seeds

1 tablespoon flax oil

1 tablespoon ground cinnamon

1 cup almond milk

In a blender, combine the spinach, apple, kiwis, flaxseed, hemp seeds, oil, cinnamon, and almond milk. Blend until smooth.

# Crunchy Green Pear Salad

MAKES 2 SERVINGS

## Salad

1 handful of arugula or watercress

2 handfuls of mixed salad greens

1 pear, cored and sliced

¼ cup walnuts

2 tablespoons crumbled goat
      cheese (optional)

## Dressing

Juice of ½ lemon

2 tablespoons olive oil

Sea salt and ground black pepper

**1.** *To make the salad:* In a large bowl, combine the arugula or watercress, greens, pear, and walnuts. Toss until thoroughly blended.

**2.** *To make the dressing:* In a small bowl, whisk together the lemon juice, oil, and sea salt and pepper to taste.

**3.** *To serve:* Drizzle the dressing over the salad, toss, and top with the goat cheese, if desired. Serve and enjoy.

# Soothing Stew for the Soul

*This stew is delicious. It takes only minutes to prepare but hours to cook, so put it in a slow cooker or on the stove top early in the day and let time work its magic.*

**MAKES 4 TO 6 SERVINGS**

2 tablespoons butter or coconut oil

1 onion, chopped

1 clove garlic, minced

1 handful of fresh sage leaves

1 handful of fresh rosemary

½ pound stewing beef, cut into small pieces

2 parsnips, peeled and quartered

4 carrots, halved

½ butternut squash, halved, seeded, and coarsely chopped

1 cup halved baby potatoes

2 tablespoons tomato puree

½ bottle red wine (optional but recommended for taste)

1 cup organic beef or vegetable stock

Ground black pepper and sea salt

1 tablespoon olive oil

**1.** Set a large pot over medium heat or preheat a slow cooker on the high setting.

**2.** Melt the butter or coconut oil, then add the onion, garlic, sage, and rosemary and cook, stirring frequently, for 2 to 3 minutes.

**3.** Add the beef, parsnips, carrots, squash, potatoes, tomato puree, wine (if using), and stock. Gently stir to combine. Season generously with pepper and a little sea salt.

**4.** Bring to a boil, cover, and reduce the heat to medium. Simmer the stew until the meat is tender (usually 3 to 4 hours). (If using a slow cooker, drop the heat to low and simmer for 8 hours, or until the meat is tender.) Stir in the olive oil just before serving.

## CHAPTER 11

# ALL-DAY FAT-BURNING SMOOTHIES AND JUICES

T he 15 smoothie and juicing recipes in this chapter are loaded with nutrients that will help reset your metabolism and facilitate fat loss. Remember, quality of ingredients—not obsession with calories—is what we're after.

I've included them here for you as substitute options for other smoothies, drinks, and even meals in the 21-day meal plan from the previous chapter. You don't have to use them, but you should certainly try them at least once because they're awesome!

You can enjoy these recipes on any of the days in this program (other than the 1-Day Fast). If you're using either the smoothie or juicing recipes on your Low-Cal Days, you may want to use them in place of your other solid meals just to keep calories lower on those days. On your 1-Day Feasts, feel free to add these liquid meals into your day whenever you need to. They provide a simple way to increase your caloric intake if you have trouble shoveling lots of solid food into your mouth.

# WHAT'S THE DIFFERENCE BETWEEN JUICES AND SMOOTHIES?

The main difference between juices and smoothies is that juices do not contain fiber (or at least have very little of it), whereas smoothies are liquid versions of whole foods, so the fiber is intact. Now, there is a slight benefit to a drink with less fiber, and that is better nutrient absorption. Fiber (aka cellulose) is the plant's "cell wall," which our human digestive tract cannot break down because we lack the enzyme cellulase. (Cows carry this enzyme, which allows them to eat copious amounts of grass without issue.)

As amazing as plant foods are for our health, the catch-22 is that sometimes we can't absorb their full spectrum of nutrients because of that damn fibrous wall. And that's where juicing comes in. Juicing strips away the fiber and leaves us with pure liquid nutrition that can easily be absorbed by our bodies. That's why juicing is very beneficial for anyone with a compromised digestive and intestinal system (i.e., almost everyone), and especially those with irritable bowel syndrome, Crohn's disease, and colitis—conditions that inhibit absorption of nutrients in the intestines.

However, when it comes to juicing, the focus should be on vegetables, not fruit, since too much fructose from juiced fruit can overload your liver and make losing weight more difficult. This problem is rare in smoothies that contain fruit because they contain the whole fruit. Thus, the protein and fiber found within a fruit help limit how much fructose leaves the stomach at a time. Just know that the recipes in this book take all of this into account so that you don't need to fuss about any of it. Cool?

# SMOOTHIE RECIPES FOR REGULAR-CAL, LOW-CAL, AND FEAST DAYS

## Green Cleaner Smoothie

1 head romaine lettuce

1 frozen banana

1 kiwifruit, unpeeled

Juice of 1 lime

1 tablespoon hemp seeds

2 tablespoons medium-chain triglyceride (MCT) oil or coconut oil

1" piece fresh ginger, peeled and grated

2 cups water

In a blender, combine the lettuce, banana, kiwi, lime juice, hemp seeds, oil, ginger, and water. Blend until smooth. Add more liquid if needed.

## Invisible Spinach Smoothie

2 large handfuls of spinach

1 handful of frozen strawberries

½ ripe banana

1 tablespoon raw cacao powder

1½ cups almond milk or hemp milk

1 tablespoon almond butter

1 teaspoon vanilla extract

1 tablespoon raw cacao nibs (optional)

In a high-speed blender, combine the spinach, strawberries, banana, cacao powder, almond or hemp milk, almond butter, and vanilla. Blend until all ingredients are completely incorporated. Pour into a glass and sprinkle with the cacao nibs, if desired.

# Glowing Skin Smoothie

½ banana
½ avocado
4 cups spinach
1 cup almond milk
Juice of ½ lemon

2 tablespoons hemp seeds
1 teaspoon vanilla extract
¼ teaspoon ground cinnamon
½ cup fresh berries

In a blender, combine the banana, avocado, spinach, almond milk, lemon juice, hemp seeds, vanilla, and cinnamon. Blend until smooth. Top with the berries. Serve and enjoy!


# Immune-Boosting Smoothie

1 handful of fresh or frozen organic
    strawberries
½ avocado
1 tablespoon chia seeds

1 tablespoon hemp seeds
1½ cups echinacea tea
1" piece fresh ginger, peeled and
    grated

In a blender, combine the strawberries, avocado, chia seeds, hemp seeds, tea, and ginger. Blend until smooth. Serve and enjoy.


# Fat Flush Detox Smoothie

1 handful of kale, stemmed
1 cup almond milk + additional
    if needed
½ frozen banana
½ ripe avocado

1 teaspoon vanilla extract
1 scoop Yuri Elkaim's Energy
    Greens
1 tablespoon chia seeds
1 tablespoon cacao nibs

In a blender, combine the kale, 1 cup of almond milk, banana, avocado, vanilla, and Energy Greens. Blend until smooth. Add more almond milk if the consistency is too thick. Top with the chia seeds and cacao nibs.

# Ginger Colada

¼ pineapple, peeled and cored

1" piece fresh ginger, peeled and grated

1 cup coconut milk

½ cup coconut water

1 teaspoon vanilla extract (optional)

In a blender, combine the pineapple, ginger, coconut milk, coconut water, and vanilla (if using). Process until smooth. Serve immediately.


# Sweet Green Almond Smoothie

2 handfuls of spinach

1 cup red grapes

1 banana

2 tablespoons almond butter

2 cups almond milk

In a blender, combine the spinach, grapes, banana, almond butter, and almond milk. Process until smooth. Serve immediately.

# SMOOTHIE RECIPES FOR LOW-CARB DAYS

## Chocolate–Peanut Butter Shake

MAKES 2 SERVINGS

1 cup almond milk + additional if
needed

2 tablespoons organic peanut
butter

1 tablespoon raw cacao powder

1 scoop protein powder

2 tablespoons full-fat coconut milk

1 teaspoon vanilla extract

5 drops liquid stevia (optional)

2 or 3 ice cubes

In a blender, combine the 1 cup of almond milk, peanut butter, cacao powder, protein powder, coconut milk, vanilla, stevia (if using), and ice cubes. Blend until smooth. Add more almond milk if too thick.

## Vanilla-Coconut Smoothie

MAKES 2 SERVINGS

1 cup coconut milk

1 cup almond milk

1 scoop vanilla protein powder

1 teaspoon vanilla extract

5 drops liquid stevia (optional)

In a blender, combine the coconut milk, almond milk, protein powder, vanilla, and stevia (if using). Blend until smooth.

# JUICE RECIPES

The following juicing recipes are suitable for any days of this plan other than the 1-Day Fasts.

## Popeye's Elixir

1 cucumber

4 handfuls of spinach

1 apple

½ lemon, peeled

In a juicer, combine the cucumber, spinach, apple, and lemon. Juice until smooth and serve.

## Red Spice

8 Swiss chard leaves

2 tomatoes

1 beet

½ small red chile pepper, seeded (wear plastic gloves when handling)

In a juicer, combine the chard, tomatoes, beet, and chile pepper. Juice until smooth and serve.

## The Super 6

1 handful of spinach

2 carrots

½ handful of parsley

1 red bell pepper

3 tomatoes

2–3 ribs celery

In a juicer, combine the spinach, carrots, parsley, bell pepper, tomatoes, and celery. Juice until smooth and serve.

# Rejuvenator

2 apples

1 cucumber

½ handful of parsley

In a juicer, combine the apples, cucumber, and parsley. Juice until smooth and serve.


# Ginger Pick-Me-Up

2 red grapefruits

1 handful of watercress
   or arugula

1" piece fresh ginger, peeled or
   unpeeled

1 pear

In a juicer, combine the grapefruits, watercress or arugula, ginger, and pear. Juice until smooth and serve.


# Red, Orange, and Green

6–8 leaves kale

4 ribs celery

2 carrots

1 beet

In a juicer, combine the kale, celery, carrots, and beet. Juice until smooth and serve.

# CHAPTER 12

# HOW TO STAY LEAN FOR LIFE

So, how many of these diet books have you read before? I'd like to believe this will be both the first and the last, but I know all too well how many people plow through countless fitness and diet texts, desperately trying to lose the weight that has made them miserable for so long. You know the routine: Every few months a friend or workmate gushes to you about a new diet or exercise that *really* works—you know, not like the other ones. You buy it, you try it, and even if you lose a few pounds, you ultimately fail.

I want you to experience what it feels like to always be in shape. This is about building fat burning into your life, making it something your body naturally does, like breathing. Can you imagine never, *ever* again groaning about a pair of pants that's too tight? What about looking forward to shopping for new clothes rather than dreading it? This can all be very real for you. I want to help you stay lean for life. The steps I've laid out for you in this book will help you lose that extra weight, but simply modifying them will allow you to do something even better: keep it off for good.

This might sound daunting, but it really shouldn't. After 21 days on this plan, you won't want to return to your old eating ways, and what's better, you'll be customizing the plan to suit your lifestyle. If you've followed the plan exactly as I've laid it out for at least 3 weeks, your body will have had enough time to start experiencing some radical health improvements, while the fat simply melts off of you like butter in a microwave oven. After the 21 days, you can start to remix the plan to your liking. Pablo Picasso once said, "Learn the rules like a pro so you can break them like an artist." Nowhere is that more true than right here.

The bigger idea at play is that you're rebooting your lifestyle. I've waited 12 chapters to tell you this, but the All-Day Fat-Burning Diet really isn't about burning fat at all—it's about learning how to truly care for the beautiful machine that is your body. You're a sleek sports car, not some busted-down old station wagon! This plan teaches you how to keep yourself running in optimum condition. Losing those pesky pounds isn't the be-all and end-all of this book; in fact, it's just the beginning of your glorious new life. Here's how easy it is to apply everything you've learned in the months and years to come.

## MODIFYING THE 5-DAY FOOD-CYCLING FORMULA

You know what's music to my ears? It's the question I'm often asked when participants complete this program: "Yuri, what do I do after 21 days?" It's a question that excites me because it means the person asking it wants to make sure she doesn't undo all the progress she's made—she's lost weight and wants to keep going or, at the very least, maintain her new body. My answer always goes one of three ways.

### *Option 1*

The first option is to continue following the 5-Day Food-Cycling Formula as it is laid out for you in this book, slightly customizing it to better suit your schedule, if needed.

For example, I first enlisted several hundred clients to go through this plan during the Christmas holidays. Almost everyone who works at my company thought I was crazy. Why on earth would I have several hundred overweight people follow a diet during the time of year when indulgent parties and feasting are the norm? The answer was quite simple: If I could help those clients lose weight and feel great during the most gluttonous, challenging time of year, just imagine what they could achieve in January, the summer, or any other time of the year when motivation is highest and circumstances are more supportive?

During that 21-day Christmas beta test, the average weight loss was 10 pounds, and a few of the women lost twice that amount. Pretty amazing, considering the final day was December 26—one day after Christmas! Many clients had work and family events that fell on the same day as their 1-Day Fast. Even Christmas Eve fell on a Low-Cal Day. So what did we do? Rather than panic, we simply shifted things around slightly. Since Christmas Day fell on their 1-Day Fast, we just swapped it with the 1-Day Feast. That's the kind of flexibility I want you to practice going forward. Yes, there will be times when you feel hungry while doing your 1-Day Fast and you might cave in and eat something after 14 hours. That's okay—don't beat yourself up over it. With consistent effort and time, your body will reset to a point where it feels absolutely normal to go a day without food.

In essence, the answer is simply this: For the first 21 days, follow the plan as closely as possible, but when that time is up, feel free to move around the 5 days as you see fit. My one suggestion is to do your best not to put your 1-Day Fast after your Low-Cal Day or Low-Carb Day. On those days, your body is likely more depleted of glycogen than usual. To follow either of those days with a 1-Day Fast would be pretty challenging for most people. Plus, we shouldn't keep your body in a low-carb or low-calorie state for too long. One day is more than enough time. That's why I've strategically placed your 1-Day Feast *before* your 1-Day Fast. That way, your body has the necessary stores to make it through your fast day.

## Option 2

The second method is to dedicate specific days of the week to a certain food-cycling day. For instance, your weekly schedule may look like the following:

| | |
|---|---|
| Monday: Regular-Cal Day | Friday: Regular-Cal Day |
| Tuesday: Low-Cal Day | Saturday: 1-Day Feast |
| Wednesday: Regular-Cal Day | Sunday: 1-Day Fast |
| Thursday: Low-Carb Day | |

Notice how all 5 days are represented during this week. The only difference is that you consistently have 3 Regular-Cal Days per week. It's a slight change, but that's totally fine. If you're someone who likes having an airtight schedule, this is definitely the option for you. Your eating and exercise get locked in place, and you don't have to ever think about them.

Personally, I find that doing a 1-Day Fast at home is too much of a challenge. It's so much easier for me to fast when I'm on the go. Why? Remember when I told you that environment will always trump will-power? That's certainly true of fast day; when you're at home, sur-rounded by food, it's much easier to take a nibble here and there without thinking twice. That said, I'm in love with my family's 1-Day Feast on Saturdays. This is when we have our "Crepe Saturdays" tradi-tion, and I love gorging on healthy crepes filled with strawberries and hazelnut chocolate spread with my kids.

## Option 3

The third option is the easiest: Just follow your gut.

My goal with this program is not to transform you into a soulless robot locked into a strict schedule. Instead, I want you to understand the nuts and bolts of food cycling so that you can make it work for you almost intuitively. The aim is that you become so attuned to your body that you don't even need to check your schedule every morning—you simply know what you should eat and how much you should exercise based on how you feel.

Let's say you have a weekend filled with a string of parties and lots of food. By the time Monday rolls around, your body should feel less inclined to eat heavier meals (assuming you have established healthy leptin-hypothalamus communication). With that in mind, you go to bed on Sunday committed to making Monday your 1-Day Fast. Almost

24 hours later, Monday night rolls around and you're ready for dinner. Satisfied, you go to bed a few hours later, expecting to roll into a Regular-Cal Day. The thing is, for whatever reason, you don't feel like eating breakfast. And that's okay—it's totally fine.

As the day progresses, you find yourself famished at lunch, so you have a huge meal. It keeps you full for most of the day, so much so that by the time dinner comes around, you opt for a small salad. By this point, you've really gone off schedule, but does it matter? Not in the slightest. If you're listening to your body, you'll know if the meal choices you're making are in alignment with your health or not. By eating only when you're hungry and stopping when you're 80 percent full, you're eating in the most sustainable fashion, the best long-term solution to staying lean for life.

However, before you can become a "body whisperer," you need to perform a full-system reset. That's why I strongly encourage you to follow the 5-Day Food-Cycling Formula in this book as closely as possible for at least 21 days. You need to experience how your body responds to a 1-Day Fast. You need to see how you feel when you limit your carb consumption for a day. You need to see how your body feels after a healthy feast. These experiences are immensely beneficial in helping you learn about true hunger, cravings, and other dieting roadblocks. Are you really hungry or are you just anxious, stressed, or bored? The discoveries you'll make, especially during your 1-Day Fast, are life-changing. This is how you end cravings for good, but you can't do it unless you first stick to the plan.

## THE 10 FAT-LOSS COMMANDMENTS

If at any point after you've successfully completed this program you find yourself falling into old habits, there's a simple way to find your way back. I call them the 10 Fat-Loss Commandments. No matter what your situation, they will help you lose fat and keep it off. If you ignore them, you will struggle for the rest of your life with yo-yoing weight fluctuations. Think of them as the core truths of the All-Day Fat-Burning Diet distilled into 10 simple rules.

### Eat Real Food

That stuff in boxes lining the shelves of the supermarket? That's not food. That edible material in tins, cans, and plastic pouches with seemingly endless lists of ingredients? That's not food either. Throughout this book I've relentlessly hit home the importance of eating real food, not man-made junk laced with chemicals. I can't state it enough. It's likely the main reason you're overweight to begin with. Eating real foods cools inflammation and reestablishes proper hormone communication, which automatically helps your body release fat it doesn't need. You stay lean without even really trying.

### Eat When You're Hungry, Stop When You're 80 Percent Full

You know the feeling—you're enjoying a meal, perhaps going for seconds or thirds, caught up in the bliss of it all. Half an hour later you feel as bloated as a beach ball. You don't need to eat until you're full, and in fact, you're probably "full" well before you think you are. By tuning in to your body, you can learn to eat only when you're truly hungry rather than when you're stressed or anxious. Better yet, you can learn to stop when you're 80 percent full. If you find yourself craving food due to stress, then find an alternative like a quick burst of activity or meditation to change your focus and reduce your stress load.

### Be Mindful and Love What You Eat

So many of us lose our way because we live our lives on autopilot, never paying attention to what we're doing or saying, thinking or feeling. This is especially true when it comes to eating. It's way too easy to eat two or three doughnuts as you drive to work in the morning, and even easier to halfheartedly devour a large order of fries while you're balancing a spreadsheet or preparing a report at work. To prevent this, never eat while you're watching TV or working at your computer. When you sit down to a meal, you should be focused on how your body feels and each bite that you take. By doing this, you're allowing yourself to feel true appreciation for the food you eat, and you'll ultimately develop a more mindful approach to eating.

## Work Out Less, Move More

One of the things I hope has really made an impression on you after reading this book is the importance of moving—not running a marathon or bench-pressing 100 pounds, mind you, but simply getting off your butt and moving around. It's really all about micromovements. Most of us spend our days trapped behind a desk, and when we're not, we're sitting in our car, on our way to and from that desk. Simply taking the stairs, taking a walk around the block, or getting up every hour or two to do a few stretches goes a long way toward keeping your muscles strong and your metabolic rate high. Keying into this movement mind-set will keep you trim.

## Build Muscle, Banish Long Cardio

Your body is often compared to a furnace, as it burns calories all day long. The general thinking is that working out accelerates this calorie burning. It does, but it's not quite as simple as that. At most, exercise accounts for only 15 percent of your total daily caloric expenditure. Your basal metabolic rate actually accounts for 70 percent of the calories you burn every single day. Thus, it makes sense to focus on increasing your basal metabolic rate, right? The only way to do that is to increase your lean body mass—aka your muscle—and that means skipping the treadmill for bodyweight or external resistance exercises. After all, we've seen how long, slow cardio destroys your body and depletes vital fat-burning hormones like triiodothyronine (T3), growth hormone, and testosterone. Your goal should be to lift heavier weights that allow you to perform only 4 to 8 reps or so. And don't forget about the power of lowering that weight slowly (eccentric contraction) to get more bang for your workout bucks.

## Set Up Your Environment to Win

The legendary Russian author and playwright Anton Chekhov once made a proclamation about writing drama that writers of all kinds still follow to this day. It's about stripping away unnecessary elements from any story in order to make it stronger. His famous words? "If you say in the first chapter that there is a rifle hanging on the wall, in the second or third chapter it absolutely must go off. If it's not going to be fired, it shouldn't be hanging there." The same can be said for those chocolate-covered pretzels in your cupboard—if you keep them around, they will get eaten. It's doubly the same for negative friends who engage in unhealthy habits—keep them around and you'll likely end up mimicking their behavior. That's just how it works. You deserve to elevate your life, so that means stripping away all the harmful elements currently polluting it. Stock your cupboards with healthy snacks and make sure you don't keep any junk in your fridge. Ditch the downer, toxic friends and join a supportive community (like the one we have on Facebook) filled with like-minded people who will support and encourage you. This is so much better than doing things on your own. Elevate it all.

## Strive for Progress, Not Perfection

This is about progress, not perfection, and like anything worth doing, it gets easier with practice. You have to go easy on yourself. If you screwed up and ate something you knew you shouldn't have, let it go and move on. If you didn't get in your workout, don't beat yourself up. Do it tomorrow. You're only human, and that means there will be times—perhaps many—when things don't go as planned. It happens, but you simply need to get back up, dust yourself off, and keep on trekking. I love the Japanese principle of *kaizen*, which essentially means "constant, never-ending improvement." A life lived in a constant state of gentle refinement is the only way to lasting success. That's what it's all about.

## Be Consistent

Key to the principle of kaizen that I just mentioned is one more familiar to us: consistency. If you eat well only occasionally, then you're not going to enjoy the slim, healthy body you want. If you aim to work out a few times this week and then stop for several months because you're sore, how are you supposed to progress toward the body of your dreams? You are much better off mastering small daily habits that, over time, will create massive change. These small daily habits can include walking, sleeping 7 to 9 hours, making a green juice, connecting with friends, laughing, doing 25 bodyweight squats, and anything else that I've laid out for you in this book. Although slightly less effective than daily habits, consistent behaviors can add up. For instance, doing a 1-Day Fast every week is a consistent behavior, even though it is not done daily. Get it? Small things done consistently will trump massive efforts that never stick.

## Keep Learning

Knowledge is power, but only if put into action. However, that action is less likely to happen if you are not first motivated by learning new and exciting ideas and strategies. You're either feeding your mind with new knowledge that helps you grow and motivates you to eat healthier and live a more active life or you're not. If you don't continue to plant new seeds in the garden of your mind, the weeds will automatically grow out of control. The mind is a precious and amazing asset, but it needs to be directed. Turn off the radio and listen to inspiring audiobooks and podcasts instead. Toss (or even burn) the newspaper and read books on health. Stop watching fake "reality" shows and go to educational seminars or watch eye-opening documentaries. You don't necessarily have to cut all these activities out of your life, but just make sure that you're engaging in behaviors that will inspire you to live your healthiest life possible. You're already off to a positive start by picking up this book.

## Be Grateful and Happy

This final commandment is a simple one, and it's truly the secret to life. Whether your goal is to become a millionaire or simply lose 20 pounds of fat and feel great about yourself, being grateful and happy is the path. No matter where you are right now, no matter what you're struggling with, you have so much to be grateful for.

It's easy to forget this when you're bombarded on a daily basis with so many worries. It takes a little work on your part, but you have to routinely tune your frequency a bit so you're more aware of the blessings in your life. When you focus on gratitude, you cannot feel sad or stressed. It's impossible. You can only feel joy, happiness, and a deep sense of appreciation for the amazing gift that is your life. When you vibrate at this higher level of awesomeness, you become an unstoppable force in the world. You feel great about yourself and thus engage in activities—like eating well and exercising—that perpetuate that feeling.

There is no right or wrong way to show gratitude. You can keep a gratitude journal, write thank-you cards to friends and family, or do anything else that keeps you in touch with the good things in your life. Here's my personal morning gratitude ritual: As soon as I open my eyes at 5:00 a.m. every morning, I scan my body and give thanks for the fact that I have all four limbs, a heart that keeps beating, an airway that brings oxygen into my body, and a body that simply works. Many people aren't so lucky.

Next, I look beside me and give thanks for my wife, Amy, the most beautiful and amazing woman in my world. Why focus on what annoys you about your loved ones? You should feel so lucky that they're still in your life.

As I get out of bed, I take a look around my bedroom, expressing gratitude for the roof and walls that keep us sheltered from the elements (especially these crazy cold Canadian winters), the blinds that darken the room so I can sleep properly, and on and on. At the end of the day, I look back over everything that has transpired since I woke up and write down all of my successes. If I'm too tired to write, I simply take a moment to play them back in my mind. I give myself a big high five for getting amazing work done, for playing with my kids, for making that green juice, for taking care of my body, and for having the opportunity to touch the lives of millions of people all around the world.

There will always be something to groan about, but I choose not to focus on those things, and I attribute whatever success I've had to this outlook. There are two sides to every coin, and which side you choose to focus on is up to you. It's always a choice. Always! You just need to be aware of your thoughts and shift them if they've veered off course. It's a universal law that you get more of what you focus on, so focus on what you're grateful for and you're likely to get more of it in your life.

## Patrick's Story

Patrick is constantly on the move, quite literally. Between traveling for work and looking after his 2-year-old son with his wife, he rarely has time to himself. Over the years, he's packed on the pounds, and his attempts at several very popular diet programs have yielded no lasting results. And yet, he found it in himself to commit to this plan and make it work.

I honestly don't know how he did it, but Patrick would wake up at 3:00 a.m. to get his workouts done before carpooling to work with his wife to get into the office by 6:30 a.m. At lunchtime, before taking lunch at his desk, he'd take a quick stroll around the block. It actually energized him. In fact, after a few weeks of doing this, he found that he had more energy by the time he got home each afternoon, allowing him more time to play with his son and also take an evening walk with his wife.

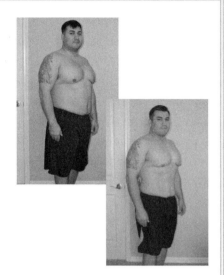

After just 2 months on the All-Day Fat-Burning Diet, Patrick lost a whopping 30 pounds and 12 inches from his waist. It sounds like a lot, but it looks like even more. The only downside, says Patrick, is that none of his clothes fit him anymore. As you can see in his before and after pictures, he's a totally new man.

And he's not finished.

Focus on problems and, *presto*, you'll get more of those as well. It's always up to you.

Are you starting to see a pattern yet? Although your weight issues are largely no fault of your own, you—and no one else—are now 100 percent responsible for turning things around. As I was finishing up this book, I drew inspiration from someone who started out just like you. His name is Patrick, and his dedication was truly inspiring.

Maybe you won't commit to waking up at 3:00 a.m. every morning, but it's my hope that over your 21 days on this program, you have a breakthrough that inspires you to make a significant, lasting change in your life as well. What started as just another diet for Patrick ended up changing his life. I know that's what you want for yourself.

I don't want you to just lose the fat that's clinging to your body, but also the stress, worries, and lack of confidence that have plagued you for so long. I want you to shed the doubt that you're capable of looking, feeling, and moving like those slender people you admire, be they at your office or on your television. It's not about comparing yourself to others, but knowing that you deserve more—you just have to reach for it. You're now armed with the know-how to not only burn fat all day, every day, but to also make each day better than the one that came before. You're already on your way.

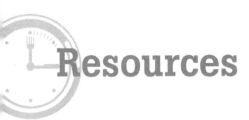

# Resources

For all of the resources mentioned throughout the book, please visit alldayfatburningdiet.com/resources. Here's a recap of what you'll find on that page.

## Workouts

Access all of the beginner, intermediate, and advanced workouts for the All-Day Fat-Burning Diet.

## Recipes

Download all of the recipes for the 21-day plan, along with beautiful photos of each.

## Facebook Group

Access the link to our readers-only All-Day Fat-Burning Diet community on Facebook.

## Extra Fat-Loss Boosters

Get all the links and recommendations for the supplements and fat-loss boosters mentioned in this book.

## Going Deeper

Want more of the nitty-gritty science behind many of the topics covered in this book? You can download that information as well on the book's resources page.

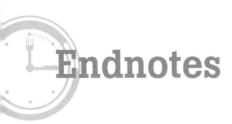

# Endnotes

## Chapter 1

[1] C. L. Ogden et al., "Mean Body Weight, Height, and Body Mass Index, United States 1960–2002," *Advance Data from Vital and Health Statistics*, no. 347 (2004).

[2] ———, "Prevalence of Childhood and Adult Obesity in the United States," *Journal of the American Medical Association* 311, no. 8 (2011–2012): 806–14.

[3] G. Corazza et al., "Celiac Disease and Alopecia Areata: Report of a New Association," *Gastroenterology* 109, no. 4 (1995): 1333–37.

[4] David MacAray, "The Man Who Saved a Billion Lives," *Huffington Post* (October 15, 2013).

[5] statista.com/statistics/237884/us-wheat-per-capita-food-use-since-2000/

[6] H. Foster-Powell and J. Brand-Miller, "International Table of Glycemic Index and Glycemic Load Values," *American Journal of Clinial Nutrition* 76, no. 1 (2002): 5–56.

[7] C. Wiseman, "Amylopectin Starch Induces Nonreversible Insulin Resistance in Rats," *Journal of Nutrition* 126, no. 2 (1996): 410–15.

[8] S. Drago et al., "Gliadin, Zonulin, and Gut Permeability: Effects on Celiac and Non-Celiac Intestinal Mucosa and Intestinal Cell Lines," *Scandinavian Journal of Gastroenterology* 41, no. 4 (2006): 408–19.

[9] J. F. Ludvigsson, S. M. Montgomery, A. Ekbom, L. Brandt, and F. Granath, "Small-Intestinal Histopathology and Mortality Risk in Celiac Disease," *Journal of the American Medical Association* 302, no. 11 (September 16, 2009): 1171–78.

[10] D. Feskanich et al., "Milk, Dietary Calcium, and Bone Fractures in Women: A 12-Year Prospective Study," *American Journal of Public Health* 87 (1997): 992–97.

[11] J. A. Kanis et al., "A Meta-Analysis of Milk Intake and Fracture Risk: Low Utility for Case Finding," *Osteoporosis International* 16 (2004): 799–804.

[12] J. Flynt, "Dairy Products Weight Loss Claims Dropped from WI Milk Marketing Board Site," on WHBL October 20, 2011 (Web: October 25, 2014).

[13] "U.S. Government Calls for End to Dairy Weight Loss Ads," *Washington Post*, May 12, 2007.

[14] C. Matthews et al., "Amount of Time Spent in Sedentary Behaviors in the United States, 2003–2004," *American Journal of Epidemiology* 167, no. 7 (2008): 875–81.

[15] M. Hamilton et al., "Exercise Physiology versus Inactivity Physiology: An Essential Concept for Understanding Lipoprotein Lipase Regulation," *Exercise and Sport Sciences Reviews* 32, no. 4 (2004): 161–66.

[16] J. Zerweth, "The Effects of Twelve Weeks of Bed Rest on Bone Histology, Biochemical Markers of Bone Turnover, and Calcium Homeostasis in Eleven Normal Subjects," *Journal of Bone and Mineral Research* 13, no. 10 (1998): 1594–1601.

[17] M. Tremblay et al., "Physiological and Health Implications of a Sedentary Lifestyle," *Applied Physiology, Nutrition, and Metabolism* 35, no. 6 (2010): 725–40.

[18] A. Patel et al., "Leisure Time Spent Sitting in Relation to Total Mortality in a Prospective Cohort of U.S. Adults," *American Journal of Epidemiology* 172, no. 4 (2010): 419–29.

[19] C. McCray and S. Agarwal, "Stress and Autoimmunity," *Immunology and Allergy Clinics of North America* 31, no. 1 (2011):1–18.

[20] R. Fry et al., "Psychological and Immunological Correlates of Acute Overtraining," *British Journal of Sports Medicine* 28, no. 4 (1994): 241–46.

[21] I. A. Lang et al., "Association of Urinary Bisphenol A Concentration with Medical Disorders and Laboratory Abnormalities in Adults," *Journal of the American Medical Association* 300, no. 11 (September 17, 2008): 1303–10.

[22] Environmental Working Group, "Study Finds Industrial Pollution Begins in the Womb," ewg.org/reports/bodyburden2/newsrelease.php

[23] L. Wallace, L. "Personal Exposures, Indoor-Outdoor Relationships, and Breath Levels of Toxic Air Pollutants Measured for 355 Persons in New Jersey," *Atmospheric Environment* 19, no. 10 (1985): 1651–61.

[24] O. A. Jones, M. L. Maguire, and J. L. Griffin, "Environmental Pollution and Diabetes: A Neglected Association," *Lancet* 371, no. 9609 (January 26, 2008): 287–88.

[25] A. M. Soto and C. Sonnenschein, "Environmental Causes of Cancer: Endocrine Disruptors as Carcinogens," *Nature Reviews Endocrinology* 6 (May 2010): 363–70.

[26] E. Montie et al., "Cytochrome P4501A1 Expression, Polychlorinated Biphenyls and Hydroxylated Metabolites, and Adipocyte Size of Bottlenose Dolphins from the Southeast United States," *Aquatic Toxicology* 86, no. 3 (2008): 397–412.

[27] H. Olsen et al., "2,3,7,8-Tetrachlorodibenzo-p-dioxin Mechanism of Action to Reduce Lipoprotein Lipase Activity in the 3T3-L1 Preadipocyte Cell Line," *Journal of Biochemical and Molecular Toxicology* 12, no. 1 (1998): 29–39.

[28] P. Phrakonkham et al., "Dietary Xenoestrogens Differentially Impair 3T3-L1 Preadipocyte Differentiation and Persistently Affect Leptin Synthesis," *Journal of Steroid Biochemistry and Molecular Biology* 110, no. 1–2 (2008): 95–103.

[29] E. Dirinck et al., "Obesity and Persistent Organic Pollutants: Possible Obesogenic Effect of Organochlorine Pesticides and Polychlorinated Biphenyls," *Obesity* 19, no. 4 (2011): 709–14.

[30] D. Mullerova et al., "Negative Association between Plasma Levels of Adiponectin and Polychlorinated Biphenyl 153 in Obese Women under Non-Energy-Restrictive Regime," *International Journal of Obesity* 32, no. 12 (2008):1875–78.

[31] E. R. Hugo et al., "Bisphenol A at Environmentally Relevant Doses Inhibits Adiponectin Release from Human Adipose Tissue Explants and Adipocytes," *Environmental Health Perspectives* 116, no. 12 (December 2008): 1642–47.

[32] F. Grün and B. Blumberg, "Environmental Obesogens: Organotins and Endocrine Disruption via Nuclear Receptor Signaling," *Endocrinology* 147, 6 Suppl. (2006): S50–55.

[33] A. Santacruz et al., "Gut Microbiota Composition Is Associated with Body Weight, Weight Gain, and Biochemical Parameters in Pregnant Women," *British Journal of Nutrition* 104, no. 1 (2010): 83–92.

[34] K. Stanhope, "Adverse Metabolic Effects of Dietary Fructose: Results from the Recent Epidemiological, Clinical, and Mechanistic Studies," *Current Opinion in Lipidology* 24, no. 3 (2013): 198–206.

[35] ———, "Consuming Fructose-Sweetened, not Glucose-Sweetened, Beverages Increases Visceral Adiposity and Lipids and Decreases Insulin Sensitivity in Overweight/Obese Humans," *Journal of Clinical Investigation* 119, no. 5 (2009): 1322–34.

[36] G. Bray, "Consumption of High-Fructose Corn Syrup in Beverages May Play a Role in the Epidemic of Obesity," *American Journal of Clinical Nutrition* 79, no. 4 (2004): 537–43.

[37] Stanhope, "Consuming Fructose-Sweetened, not Glucose-Sweetened, Beverages," 1322–34.

[38] T. Nakagawa, "A Causal Role for Uric Acid in Fructose-Induced Metabolic Syndrome," *American Journal of Physiology—Renal Physiology* 290, no. 3 (2006): F625–31.

[39] X. Ouyang, "Fructose Consumption as a Risk Factor for Non-Alcoholic Fatty Liver Disease," *Journal of Hepatology* 48, no. 6 (2008): 993–99.

[40] H. Basciano et al., "Fructose, Insulin Resistance, and Metabolic Dyslipidemia," *Nutrition and Metabolism* 2 (February 2005): 5.

[41] K. Page et al., "Effects of Fructose vs. Glucose on Regional Cerebral Blood Flow in Brain Regions Involved with Appetite and Reward Pathways," *Journal of the American Medical Association* 309, no. 1 (2013): 63–70.

[42] A. Shapiro, "Fructose-Induced Leptin Resistance Exacerbates Weight Gain in Response to Subsequent High-Fat Feeding," *American Journal of Physiology—Regulatory, Integrative, and Comparative Physiology* 295, no. 5 (2008): R1370–75.

[43] http://www.odwalla.com/products/smoothies/original-superfood

[44] Centers for Disease Control and Prevention (CDC), "Trends in Intake of Energy and Macronutrients—United States, 1971–2000," *Morbidity and Mortality Weekly Report* 53, no. 4 (2004): 80.

[45] E. Ford and W. Dietz, "Trends in Energy Intake among Adults in the United States: Findings from NHANES," *American Journal of Clinical Nutrition* 97, no. 4 (April 2013): 848–53.

[46] Q. Zhou et al., "Dopamine-Deficient Mice Are Severely Hypoactive, Adipsic, and Aphagic," *Cell* 83 (1995): 1197–1209.

[47] M. Yeomans et al., "Palatability: Response to Nutritional Need or Need-Free Stimulation of Appetite?" *British Journal of Nutrition* 92, Suppl. S1 (2004): S3–14.

[48] R. J. Johnson et al., "Potential Role of Sugar (Fructose) in the Epidemic of Hypertension, Obesity and the Metabolic Syndrome, Diabetes, Kidney Disease, and Cardiovascular Disease," *American Journal of Clinical Nutrition* 86, no. 4 (October 2007): 899–906.

[49]ers.usda.gov/data-products/food-expenditures.aspx

[50]fmi.org/research-resources

[51] K. Chen, "Induction of Leptin Resistance through Direct Interaction of C-Reactive Protein with Leptin," *Nature Medicine* 12 (2006): 425–32.

[52] A. Shapiro, "Fructose-Induced Leptin Resistance Exacerbates Weight Gain in Response to Subsequent High-Fat Feeding," *Integrative and Comparative Physiology* 295, no. 5 (November 1, 2008): R1370–75.

[53] J. M. de Castro and E. M. Brewer, "The Amount Eaten in Meals by Humans Is a Power Function of the Number of People Present," *Physiology and Behavior* 51, no. 1 (1992): 121.

[54] J. Danguir and S. Nicolaidis, "Dependence of Sleep on Nutrients' Availability," *Physiology and Behavior* 22, no. 4 (1979): 735–40.

[55] C. A. Everson, B. M. Bergmann, and A. Rechtschaffen, "Sleep Deprivation in the Rat: III. Total Sleep Deprivation," *Sleep* 12, no. 1 (1989): 13–21.

[56] D. Kripke, R. Simons, L. Garfinkel et al., "Short and Long Sleep and Sleeping Pills. Is Increased Mortality Associated?" *Archives of General Psychiatry* 36, no. 1 (1979): 103–16.

[57] National Sleep Foundation, "Sleep in America Poll, 2001-2002," Washington, DC.

## Chapter 2

[1] A. Barletta, G. et al., *Journal of Endocrinological Investigation* 3 (1980): 293–96.

[2] F. Goglia, G. Liverini, T. De Leo, and A. Barletta, "Thyroid State and Mitochondrial Population during Cold Exposure," *Pflügers Archiv-European Journal of Physiology* 396, no. 1 (1983): 49–53.

[3] H. Sul and D. Wang, "Nutritional and Hormonal Regulation of Enzymes in Fat Synthesis: Studies of Fatty Acid Synthase and Mitochondrial Glycerol-3-Phosphate Acultransferase Gene Transcription," *Annual Review of Nutrition* 18 (1998): 331–51.

[4] G. J. Canaris, N. R. Manowitz, G. Mayor, and E. C. Ridgway, "The Colorado Thyroid Disease Prevalence Study," *Archives of Internal Medicine* 160 (2000): 526–34.

[5] T. Teixeira, "Potential Mechanisms for the Emerging Link between Obesity and Increased Intestinal Permeability," *Nutrition Research* 32, no. 9 (September 2012): 637–47.

[6] F. Grün and B. Blumberg, "Environmental Obesogens: Organotins and Endocrine Disruption via Nuclear Receptor Signaling," *Endocrinology* 147, no. 6 Suppl. (2006): S50–55.

[7] A. Shapiro, W. Mu, C. Roncal, K. Y. Cheng, R. J. Johnson, and P. J. Scarpace, "Fructose-Induced Leptin Resistance Exacerbates Weight Gain in Response to Subsequent High-Fat Feeding," *Amercian Journal of Physiology—Regulatory, Integrative, and Comparative Physiology* 295, no. 5 (2008): R1370–75.

## Chapter 3

[1] R. R. Wing and R. W. Jeffery, "Benefits of Recruiting Participants with Friends and Increasing Social Support for Weight Loss and Maintenance," *Journal of Consulting and Clinical Psychology* 7, no. 1 (1999): 132–38.

[2] K. Hwang et al., "Social Support in an Internet Weight Loss Community," *International Journal of Medical Informatics* 79, no. 1 (2010): 5–13.

[3] M. Gailliot et al., "Self-Control Relies on Glucose as a Limited Energy Source: Willpower Is More Than a Metaphor," *Journal of Personality and Social Psychology* 92, no. 2 (2007): 325–36.

## Chapter 4

[1] Ancel Keys, *Seven Countries: A Multivariate Analysis of Death and Coronary Heart Disease* (Cambridge, MA: Harvard University Press, 1980).

[2] R. Chowdhury et al., "Association of Dietary, Circulating, and Supplement Fatty Acids with Coronary Risk: A Systematic Review and Meta-Analysis," *Annals of Internal Medicine* 160, no. 6 (2014): 398–406.

[3] J. F. Mauger et al., "Effect of Different Forms of Dietary Hydrogenated Fats on LDL Particle Size," *American Journal of Clinical Nutrition* 78, no. 3 (2003): 370–75.

[4] R. Khanal, "Potential Health Benefits of Conjugated Linoleic Acid (CLA): A Review," *Asian-Australasian Journal of Animal Sciences* 17, no. 9 (2004): 1315–28.

[5] Z. Gao et al., "Butyrate Improves Insulin Sensitivity and Increases Energy Expenditure in Mice," *Diabetes* 58, no. 7 (2009): 1509–17.

[6] A. Christianson, *The Adrenal Reset Diet* (New York: Harmony Books, 2014).

[7] S. W. Souci, E. Fachmann, and H. Kraut, *Food Composition and Nutrition Tables* (Stuttgart, Germany: Medpharm Scientific Publishers, 2008).

[8] A. Afshin, "Consumption of Nuts and Legumes and Risk of Incident Ischemic Heart Disease, Stroke, and Diabetes: A Systematic Review and Meta-Analysis," *American Journal of Clinical Nutrition* 100, no. 1 (July 1, 2014): 278–88.

[9] A. Salehi-Abargouei et al., "Effects of Non-Soy Legume Consumption on C-Reactive Protein: A Systematic Review and Meta-Analysis," *Nutrition* 31, no. 5 (2015): 631–39.

[10] H. Hermsdorff, "A Legume-Based Hypocaloric Diet Reduces Proinflammatory Status and Improves Metabolic Features in Overweight/Obese Subjects," *European Journal of Nutrition* 50, no. 1 (2011): 61–69.

[11] D. Birt et al., "Resistant Starch: Promise for Improving Human Health," *Advances in Nutrition* 4, no. 6 (2013): 587–601.

[12] M. Säemann et al., "Anti-Inflammatory Effects of Sodium Butyrate on Human Monocytes: Potent Inhibition of IL-12 and Up-Regulation of IL-10 Production," *FASEB Journal* 14, no. 15 (December 2000): 2380–82.

[13] O. Kanauchi et al., "Butyrate from Bacterial Fermentation of Germinated Barley Foodstuff Preserves Intestinal Barrier Function in Experimental Colitis in the Rat Model," *Journal of Gastroenterology and Hepatology* 14, no. 9 (1999): 880–88.

[14] D. Robertson et al., "Insulin-Sensitizing Effects of Dietary Resistant Starch and Effects on Skeletal Muscle and Adipose Tissue Metabolism," *American Journal of Clinical Nutrition* 82, no. 3 (2005): 559–67.

## Chapter 5

[1] C. S. Johnston et al., "Ketogenic Low-Carbohydrate Diets Have No Metabolic Advantage over Nonketogenic Low-Carbohydrate Diets," *American Journl of Clinical Nutrition* 83, no. 5 (May 2006): 1055–61.

[2] S. Soenen et al., "Relatively High-Protein or 'Low-Carb' Energy-Restricted Diets for Body Weight Loss and Body Weight Maintenance?" *Physiology & Behavior* 107, no. 3 (October 10, 2012): 374–80.

[3] A. Raben, I. Macdonald, and A. Astrup, "Replacement of Dietary Fat by Sucrose or Starch: Effects on 14 d ad libitum Energy Intake, Energy Expenditure and Body Weight in Formerly Obese and Never-Obese Subjects," *International Journal of Obesity and Related Metabolic Disorders* 21, no. 10 (1997): 846–59.

[4] M. Mattson and R. Wan, "Beneficial Effects of Intermittent Fasting and Caloric Restriction on the Cardiovascular and Cerebrovascular Systems," *Journal of Nutritional Biochemistry* 16, no. 3 (2005): 129–37.

[5] A. Muller et al., "Ghrelin Drives GH Secretion during Fasting in Man," *European Journal of Endocrinology* 146, no. 2 (2002): 203–7.

## Chapter 6

[1] S. Haskins, "4 Reasons Why Diets Don't Work," retrieved from health.usnews.com /health-news/blogs/eat-run/2015/01/21/4-reasons-why-diets-dont-work (Jan. 21, 2015).

[2] Boston Medical Center, "Nutrition and Weight Management," retrieved from bmc.org /nutritionweight/services/weightmanagement.htm (2014).

[3] P. Schnohr, J. H. O'Keefe, J. L. Marott, P. Lange, and G. B. Jensen, "Dose of Jogging and Long-Term Mortality: The Copenhagen City Heart Study," *Journal of the American College of Cardiology* 65, no. 5 (2015): 411–19.

[4] J. Talanian et al., "Two Weeks of High-Intensity Aerobic Interval Training Increases the Capacity for Fat Oxidation during Exercise in Women," *Journal of Applied Physiology* 102, no. 4 (April 2007): 1439–47.

[5] M. Gibala and S. McGee, "Metabolic Adaptations to Short-Term High-Intensity Interval Training: A Little Pain for a Lot of Gain?" *Exercise and Sport Sciences Reviews* 36, no. 2 (2008): 58–63.

[6] D. Malatesta et al., "Effect of High-Intensity Interval Exercise on Lipid Oxidation during Postexercise Recovery," *Medicine and Science in Sports and Exercise (Journal Impact Factor: 4.48)* 41, no. 2 (February 2009): 364–74.

[7] L. Deldicque, K. De Bock, M. Maris et al., "Increased p70s6k Phosphorylation during Intake of a Protein-Carbohydrate Drink Following Resistance Exercise in the Fasted State," *European Journal of Applied Physiology* 108, no. 4 (2009): 791–800.

[8] L. Baylor and A. Hackney, "Resting Thyroid and Leptin Hormone Changes in Women Following Intense, Prolonged Exercise Training," *European Journal of Applied Physiology* 88, no. 4–5 (2003): 480–84. Epub 2002 Nov 22.

[9] A. Hackney, "Endurance Training and Testosterone Levels," *Sports Medicine* 8, no. 2 (1989): 117–27.

[10] H. Cakir-Atabek et al., "Effects of Different Resistance Training Intensity on Indices of Oxidative Stress," *Journal of Strength and Conditioning Research* 24, no. 9 (2010): 2491–98.

[11] K. Sonneville and S. Gortmaker, "Total Energy Intake, Adolescent Discretionary Behaviors and the Energy Gap," *International Journal of Obesity* 32, Suppl. 6 (2008): S19–27.

[12] R. Fry et al., "Psychological and Immunological Correlates of Acute Overtraining," *British Journal of Sports Medicine* 28, no. 4 (1994): 241–46.

[13] T. Akerström and B. Pedersen, "Strategies to Enhance Immune Function for Marathon Runners: What Can Be Done?" *Sports Medicine* 37, no. 4–5 (2007): 416–19.

[14] Jeffrey Warren King, "A Comparison of the Effects of Interval Training vs. Continuous Training on Weight Loss and Body Composition in Obese Pre-Menopausal Women." Electronic Theses and Dissertations. Paper 123 (2001). dc.etsu.edu/etd/123.

[15] M. J. Gibala and J. P. Little, "Just HIT It! A Time-Efficient Exercise Strategy to Improve Muscle Insulin Sensitivity," *Journal of Physiology* 588, no. 18 (2010): 3341–42.

[16] M. J. Gibala, J. P. Little, M. V. Essen et al., "Short-Term Sprint Interval versus Traditional Endurance Training: Similar Initial Adaptations in Human Skeletal Muscle and Exercise Performance," *Journal of Physiology* 575, no. 3 (2006): 901–11.

[17] J. P. Little, A. Safdar, G. P. Wilkin, M. A. Ranopolsky, and M. J. Gibala, "A Practical Model of Low-Volume High-Intensity Interval Training Induces Mitochondrial Biogenesis in Human Skeletal Muscle: Potential Mechanisms," *Journal of Physiology* 588, no. 6 (2010): 1011–22.

[18] I. Tabata, K. Nishimura, M. Kouzaki et al., "Effects of Moderate-Intensity Endurance and High-Intensity Intermittent Training on Anaerobic Capacity and Max VO2," *Medicine and Science in Sports and Exercise* 28, no. 10 (October 1996): 1327–30.

[19] D. L. Elliot, L. Goldberg, and K. S. Kuehl, "Effects of Resistance Training on Excess Post-Exercise O2 Consumption," *Journal of Strength and Conditioning Research* 6, no. 2 (1992): 77–81.

[20] E. Murphy and R. Schwarzkopf, "Effects of Standard Set and Circuit Weight Training on Excess Post-Exercise Oxygen Consumption," *Journal of Strength and Conditioning Research* 6, no. 2 (1992): 66–124.

[21] N. Moller, O. Schmitz, N. Porksen, J. Moller, and J. O. Jorgenson, "Dose-Response Studies on the Metabolic Effects of a Growth Hormone Pulse in Humans," *Metabolism* 41, no. 2 (1992): 172–75.

[22] Murphy and Schwarzkopf, "Effects of Standard Set and Circuit Weight Training," 66–124.

[23] L. Heden, C. Lox, P. Rose, S. Reid, and E. P. Kirk, "One Set Resistance Training Elevates Energy Expenditure for 72 Hours Similar to Three Sets," *European Journal of Applied Physiology* 111, no. 3 (2011): 477–84.

[24] A.Bubbico and L. Kravitz, "Eccentric Training," *IDEA Fitness Journal* 7, no. 10 (October 2010).

[25] ibid.

[26] E. Colliander and P. Tesch, "Effects of Eccentric and Concentric Muscle Actions in Resistance Training," *Acta Physiologica Scandinavica* 140, no. 1 (September 1990): 31–39.

[27] R. Carpinelli and R. Otto, "Strength Training. Single versus Multiple Sets," *Sports Medicine* 26, no. 2 (August 1998): 73–84.

[28] J. Burt et al., "A Comparison of Once versus Twice per Week Training on Leg Press Strength in Women," *Journal of Sports Medicine and Physical Fitness* 47, no. 1 (2007): 13–17.

[29] R. Pratley et al., "Strength Training Increases Resting Metabolic Rate and Norepinephrine Levels in Healthy 50- to 65-Yr-Old Men," *Journal of Applied Physiology* 76, no. 1 (1994): 133–37.

[30] J. Farthing and P. Chilibeck, "The Effects of Eccentric and Concentric Training at Different Velocities on Muscle Hypertrophy," *European Journal of Applied Physiology* 89, no. 6 (2003): 578–86. Epub 2003 May 17.

[31] Y. Izumiya et al., "Fast/Glycolytic Muscle Fiber Growth Reduces Fat Mass and Improves Metabolic Parameters in Obese Mice," *Cell Metabolism* 7, no. 2 (2008): 159–72.

## Chapter 7

[1] R. Bahr, "Sports Medicine," *British Medical Journal* 323, no. 7308 (2001): 328–31.

[2] A. Rosengren and L. Wilhelmsen, "Physical Activity Protects against Coronary Death and Deaths from All Causes in Middle-Aged Men. Evidence from a 20-Year Follow-Up of the Primary Prevention Study in Göteborg," *Annals of Epidemiology* 7, no. 1 (1997): 69–75.

[3] A. Gergley, "Acute Effect of Passive Static Stretching on Lower-Body Strength in Moderately Trained Men," *Journal of Strength and Conditioning Research* 27, no. 4 (April 2013): 973–77.

[4] L. Simic et al., "Does Pre-Exercise Static Stretching Inhibit Maximal Muscular Performance? A Meta-Analytical Review," *Scandinavian Journal of Medicine and Science in Sports* 23, no. 2 (March 2013): 131–48.

[5] I. Shrier, "Stretching before Exercise Does Not Reduce the Risk of Local Muscle Injury: A Critical Review of the Clinical and Basic Science Literature," *Clinical Journal of Sport Medicine* 9, no. 4 (1999): 221–27.

[6] J. Vaile, S. Halson, N. Gill, and B. Dawson, "Effect of Hydrotherapy on the Signs and Symptoms of Delayed Onset Muscle Soreness," *European Journal of Applied Physiology* 102, no. 4 (2008): 447–55.

[7] A. Mohr et al., "Effect of Foam Rolling and Static Stretching on Passive Hip-Flexion Range of Motion," *Journal of Sport Rehabilitation* 23, no. 4 (2014): 296–99.

[8] B. S. Kawamoto, E. J. Drinkwater, D. G. Behm, and C. Duane, "Foam Rolling for Delayed-Onset Muscle Soreness and Recovery of Dynamic Performance Measures," *Journal of Athletic Training* 50, no. 1 (2015): 5–13.

## Chapter 8

[1] S. S. Kraus and L. A. Rabin, "Sleep America: Managing the Crisis of Adult Chronic Insomnia and Associated Conditions," *Journal of Affective Disorders* 138, no. 3 (2012): 192–212.

[2] A. M. Chang, J. Aeschbach, J. F. Duffy, and C. A. Czeisler, "Evening Use of Light-Emitting eReaders Negatively Affects Sleep, Circadian Timing, and Next-Morning Alertness," *Proceedings of the National Academy of Sciences* 112, no. 4 (December 22, 2014): 1232–37.

[3] National Sleep Foundation, "How Much Sleep Do We Really Need?" n.d. retrieved April 16, 2012.

[4] Rhonda Rowland (15 February 2002), "Experts Challenge Study Linking Sleep, Life Span," CNN, retrieved October 29, 2013.

[5] S. R. Patel, N. T. Ayas, M. R. Malhotra, D. P. White, E. S. Schernhammer, F. E. Speizer, M. J. Stampfer, and F. B. Hu, "A Prospective Study of Sleep Duration and Mortality Risk in Women," *Sleep* 27, no. 3 (May 2004): 440–44.

[6] S. R. Patel, A. Malhotra, D. J. Gottlieb, D. P. White, and F. B. Hu, "Correlates of Long Sleep Duration," *Sleep* 29, no. 7 (July 2006): 881–89. PMC 3500381. PMID 16895254.; cf. M. R. Irwin and M. Ziegler, "Sleep Deprivation Potentiates Activation of Cardiovascular and Catecholamine Responses in Abstinent Alcoholics," *Hypertension* 45, no. 2 (February 2005): 252–57.

[7] J. K. Wyatt, A. Ritz-De Cecco, C. A. Czeisler, and D. J. Dijk, "Circadian Temperature and Melatonin Rhythms, Sleep, and Neurobehavioral Function in Humans Living on a 20-h Day," *American Journal of Physiology* 277, no. 4 (October 1, 1999): R1152–63.

[8] C. Eastman, "High-Intensity Light for Circadian Adaptation to a 12-h Shift of the Sleep Schedule," *American Journal of Physiology—Regulatory, Integrative, and Comparative Physiology* 263, no. 2 (1992): R428–36.

[9] K. Sharkey, "Effects of an Advanced Sleep Schedule and Morning Short Wavelength Light Exposure on Circadian Phase in Young Adults with Late Sleep Schedules," *Sleep Medicine* 12, no. 7 (2011): 685–92.

[10] H. Burgess and C. Eastman, "Early versus Late Bedtimes Phase Shift the Human Dim Light Melatonin Rhythm despite a Fixed Morning Lights on Time," *Neuroscience Letters* 356, no. 2 (2004): 115–18.

[11] J. P. Chaput et al., "The Association between Sleep Duration and Weight Gain in Adults: A 6-Year Prospective Study from the Quebec Family Study," *Sleep* 31, no. 4 (2008): 517–23.

[12] L. Neilsen et al., "Short Sleep Duration as a Possible Cause of Obesity: Critical Analysis of the Epidemiological Evidence," *Obesity Reviews* 12, no. 2 (2010): 78–92.

[13] M. Münch et al., "Wavelength-Dependent Effects of Evening Light Exposure on Sleep Architecture and Sleep EEG Power Density in Men," *American Journal of Physiology—Regulatory, Integrative, and Comparative Physiology* 290, no. 5 (2006): R1421–28.

[14] R. Wallace, "Physiological Effects of Transcendental Meditation," *Revista Brasileira de Medicina do Esporte* 27, no. 8 (1970): 397–401.

[15] P. N. Ravindra, S. Sulekha, T. N. Sathyaprabha, N. Pradhan, T. R. Raju, and B. M. Kutty, "Practitioners of Vipassana Meditation Exhibit Enhanced Slow Wave Sleep and REM Sleep States across Different Age Groups," *Sleep and Biological Rhythms* 8, no. 1 (2010): 34–41.

[16] S. Wu and P. Lo, "Inward-Attention Meditation Increases Parasympathetic Activity: A Study Based on Heart Rate Variability," *Biomed Research International* 29, no. 5 (2008): 245–50.

[17] R. Jevning, "The Transcendental Meditation Technique, Adrenocortical Activity, and Implications for Stress," *Experientia* 34, no. 5 (1978): 618–19.

[18] C. Maclean et al., "Effects of the Transcendental Meditation Program on Adaptive Mechanisms: Changes in Hormone Levels and Responses to Stress after 4 Months of Practice," *Psychoneuroendocrinology* 22, no. 4 (1997): 277–95.

[19] G. A. Tooley et al., "Acute Increases in Night-Time Plasma Melatonin Levels Following a Period of Meditation," *Biological Psychology* 53, no. 1 (2000): 69–78.

[20] R. Freedman and J. Papsdorf, "Biofeedback and Progressive Relaxation Treatment of Sleep-Onset Insomnia," *Biofeedback and Self-Regulation* 1, no. 3 (1976): 253–71.

[21] A. Lewy, "Antidepressant and Circadian Phase-Shifting Effects of Light," *Science* 235, no. 4786 (1987): 352–54.

[22] "Effects of Diet on Tryptophan (Trp) Uptake and the Central Nervous System," adapted from A. Grimmett and M. N. Sillence, "Calmatives for the Excitable Horse: A Review of L-Tryptophan," *Veterinary Journal* 170, no. 1 (2005): 24–32.

[23] J. D. Fernstrom and R. J. Wurtman, "Brain Serotonin Content: Physiological Dependence on Plasma Tryptophan Levels," *Science* 173, no. 3992 (1971): 149–52.

[24] G. K. Zammit, A. Kolevzon, M. Fauci, R. Shindledecker, and S. Ackerman, "Postprandial Sleep in Healthy Men," *Sleep* 18, no. 4 (1995): 229–31.

[25] S. Youngstedt et al., "The Effects of Acute Exercise on Sleep: A Quantitative Synthesis," *Sleep* 20, no. 3 (March 1997): 203–14.

[26] H. Chtourou et al., "Effect of Time-of-Day of Aerobic Maximal Exercise on the Sleep Quality of Trained Subjects," *Biological Rhythm Research* 43, no. 3 (2012): 323–30.

## *Chapter 9*

[1] P. La Bounty et al., "International Society of Sports Nutrition Position Stand: Meal Frequency," *Journal of the International Society of Sports Nutrition* 8, no. 4 (2011).

[2] F. A. Scheer, M. F. Hilton, C. S. Mantzoros, and S. A. Shea, "Adverse Metabolic and Cardiovascular Consequences of Circadian Misalignment," *Proceedings of the National Academy of Sciences* 106, no. 11 (2009): 4453–58.

# Index

Boldface page references indicate illustrations. <u>Underscored</u> references indicate boxed text.

# I

Ice, 173
Immune system
  harm from overtraining, 18–19,
    132–33
  hyperactive, 48
Inflammation
  after deep-tissue work, 177
  cortisol increase with, 39, 40, 47
  C-reactive protein as marker of,
    83
  decrease with
    butyrate, 79, 85
    "clean and lean" foods, 75
    cold therapy, 173
    legumes, 83
    resistant starch, 85
  sources, 7–16
    dairy producers, 13–16
    gluten, 10–12
    insulin, 39, 40
    leaky gut, 47
    leptin resistance, 33, 49
    lipopolysaccharides (LPS),
      46–47
    toxins, 20
    trans fats, 78
    wheat, 8–13
  stress, 39, 47
Injury, 163–64, 168, 171, 175–76
Insulin, 38–40
  blood sugar spikes and, 10
  butyrate effects on levels and sensitivity
    to, 79
  decrease with
    intermittent fasting, 102
    resistant starch, 86
  effect of eating at bedtime, 207
  as fat-storage hormone, 24
  fluctuations, 40
  impairment of weight loss, 40
Insulin resistance, 10–11, 23, 25, 39, 46,
    79, 209
Intensity of exercise
  fat burning, 126, 134, 136
  in LIFT method, 118–19
Interval training
  benefits of, 121
  speed bursts, 121–23
  warmup for, 124
Intestines
  gluten effect on lining, 11
  permeability, 13, 22, 45–48, 85
Iron, 82

# J

Jet lag, 181
Juices/juicing
  benefits, 274
  downsides of, 26, 274
  green, 110–11
  ingredients, 26–27
  recipes, 279–80
    Ginger Pick-Me-Up, 280
    Popeye's Elixir, 279
    Red, Orange, and Green, 280
    Red Spice, 279
    Rejuvenator, 280
    The Super 6, 279
Junk food, 50, 67–68, 74–75, 97, 286

# K

Kaizen, 288
Ketogenic diet, 91

# L

Lactase, 13
Lactic acid, 173
Lactose, 13, 77
Lactose intolerance, 13
Large neutral amino acids, 193–94
Law of attraction, 60, 68
LDL (low-density lipoprotein) cholesterol,
    23, 78, 91
Leafy greens, 93
Leaky gut, 13, 22, 41, 45–48, 85
Learning, 288
Legumes, 10, 82–83, 100
Length of workout, 117–18
Leptin, 49–51
  carbohydrate influence on, 99
  cortisol effect on, 41
  decrease with
    cardio exercise, 131
    disrupted circadian rhythm, 209
  insulin link to, 40
  role in body, 20, 33
  sleep effect on, 35
Leptin resistance, 22, 26, 33–34,
    49–50
LIFT method, 18, 115, 117–20
  frequency, 119–20
  intensity, 118–19
  length, 117–18
  tempo, 120

# M

Metabolic rate *(cont.)*
    increasing with workout intensity,
        118–19
    postworkout, 137
    thyroid gland role in, 43
Microbiome, 21–23
Micromovement challenge, 167
Micromovements, 166–68, 287
Milk, 13–16, 76–77
Mindful approach to eating, 286
Minicircuits, 136
Mitochondria, 43
Mobility exercises, 168
Molecular mimicry, 22
Mood improvement with morning light, 192
Muscle(s)
    building, 287
    bulking up, 150
    decrease with
        age, 136
        endurance training, 131
    easing with deep-tissue work, 174–77
    increasing lean, 116–17
    tight, 174
Muscle fibers, 147–49
Myostatin, 150

# N

NatureBright's SunTouch Plus Light, 193
Neurotransmitters
    sleep influenced by, 193
    thyroid gland and, 44
New Year's resolutions, 57–58
Nonalcoholic fatty liver disease, 25
Norepinephrine, 102
Nuts, 100

# O

Obesity
    calorie consumption increase, 28
    decreased risk with physically active
        leisure time, 166
    increase with
        intestinal permeability, 46
        short sleep duration, 186
    insulin resistance, 25
    overeating as self-sustaining habit, 33
    statistics on, 4
    wheat's contribution to, 8
1-Day Fast, 101–8
    in 21-day meal plan, 230, 246, 258, 270
    exercise guidelines, 108, 213
    food guidelines, 108, 213
    rest or active recovery, 143
    scheduling, 283–85

serving sizes, 202–4
1-Day Feast, 95–101
    exercise, 101, 129–42, 213
    foods, 99–101, 212
    placement before 1-Day Fast, 283
    recipes, 227–29, 243–45, 255–57,
        267–69
        Brown Rice with Steamed Greens,
            Roasted Veggies, and Avocado,
            268
        Cherry Protein Smoothie, 256
        Choco-Coco-Oatmeal Pancakes, 257
        Fat Flush Detox Smoothie, 276
        Ginger Colada, 277
        Glowing Skin Smoothie, 276
        Gluten-Free Banana-Coconut
            Pancakes, 243
        Green Almond Smoothie, 227
        Green Cleaner Smoothie, 275
        Immune-Boosting Smoothie, 276
        Invisible Spinach Smoothie, 275
        Mushroom Chicken Pasta, 269
        Protein Lover's Casserole, 255
        Quinoa Chili, 228
        Red Lentil Curry-Covered Rice, 245
        Salmon Teriyaki Rice Bowl, 244
        Seared Halibut, Peach Salsa, and
            Cooled Potatoes, 229
        Strawberry-Vanilla-Oat Shake, 267
        Sweet Green Almond Smoothie, 277
    serving sizes, 202–4, 212
Osteoporosis, 15, 135
Overtraining, 18–19, 119, 133, 165
Overweight individuals
    gut bacteria composition, 22–23
    health risks, 4
    insulin resistance, 39
Oxidative damage, 102, 131

# P

Pectoralis muscles, 165
Peptide YY3-36, 31
Philips Wake-Up Light, 192
Phosphatidylserine, 83
Phosphorus, in dairy products, 14
Phytic acid, 82
Planning, 62–63
Plantains, 85
Portion size, 108–12, 202–4
Posture, 64
Postworkout meals, 127–28
Potatoes, 85
Potato starch, 85–86
Prebiotic, 85
Preparation, 62–63
Processed foods, 12, 28, 31–32, 74